DATA DRIVEN HEALTH

How I Hacked My Health, Fixed Chronic Illnesses, and Survived
Emergency Surgery with DIY Open Source Tools

First Edition

Roberto Rosario

robertorosario.com

First Edition

Identifiers: ISBN 979-8-9991780-0-8 (paperback) | ISBN 979-8-9991780-1-5 (ebook) | ISBN 979-8-9991780-2-2 (hardcover)

Classifiers: DDC 362.1

TABLE OF CONTENTS

DEDICATION

To the three people who make every day worth writing about. My wife Lorena, my partner in every sense of the word; to Cesare, who brings laughter and wonder into our lives; and to Brandon, whose growth and accomplishments fill me with pride. This book is a small token of my love for you all.

DISCLAIMER

The information presented herein reflects the author's interpretations and should not be construed as medical advice, a diagnosis, or a treatment plan.

This book chronicles the author's journey through health, healing, self-experimentation, and spiritual exploration. It is based on lived experience, independent research, and reflection and includes interpretations of scientific and medical literature. However, this content is not intended to serve as medical advice, nor should it be used as a substitute for professional consultation, diagnosis, or treatment.

While references to studies and academic articles are included to provide context and support the author's perspective, these citations do not imply a consensus view within the medical community, nor do they guarantee clinical validation or applicability to individual health situations. The information presented may contain inaccuracies or reflect outdated knowledge, and conclusions may not align with prevailing scientific understanding.

Readers are encouraged to consult sources and qualified healthcare professionals for the most current and reliable information. The conclusions drawn within this book are inherently personal and may be incomplete, evolving, or subject to error.

The practices discussed, including but not limited to dietary experimentation, fasting, supplementation, spiritual disciplines, and biohacking techniques, carry inherent risks. What works for one individual may be ineffective or even harmful for another. Therefore, it is strongly advised to consult a qualified healthcare professional before initiating any health-related protocol, particularly if you have a pre-existing medical condition, are pregnant or nursing, or are taking prescription medications.

This book aims to foster self-reflection, body awareness, and informed exploration; however, it is not a guide for treatment or diagnosis. The goal is to stimulate critical thinking and personal responsibility in the pursuit of wellness, not to replace conventional medical care or spiritual guidance from qualified professionals.

The author and publisher expressly disclaim all liability for any adverse effects, injuries, or damages resulting from the application of information contained within this book. All actions taken based on this information are solely at the reader's discretion and risk. This publication does not establish a doctor-patient relationship.

In all matters related to health, healing, and transformation, whether physical, emotional, or spiritual, we urge readers to proceed with discernment, humility, and the support of qualified professionals as needed.

If you have or suspect you may have a medical condition, consult your healthcare provider promptly. Do not disregard professional medical advice or delay seeking it due to information encountered in this book.

1

INTRODUCTION

My journey

"Accept whatever comes to you woven in the pattern of your destiny, for what could more aptly fit your needs?" - *Marcus Aurelius, Meditations*

I should have died, twice.

The first time, in 2016, when my heart, despite years of martial arts training and "clean eating", **screamed** at me that something was **deeply broken**.

The second time, in 2025, when a routine appendectomy turned into a life-threatening emergency requiring the removal of parts of my intestines.

Both times, I walked away **stronger, faster,** and **healthier**.

Not just because of answered prayers or luck smiled upon me.

But because **I hacked my health like a software system**.

If you've ever felt like you're following every rule, eating the "right" foods, exercising regularly, and listening to doctors, yet something still feels off, then **this book might be for you**.

Maybe it's brain fog, irritable bowel syndrome, fatigue, or weight you can't lose. Strange symptoms that come and go. Tests that return "normal" even as you feel far from it. I've been there too.

In 2016, a life-threatening cardiac event left me **bedridden** and **frustrated** with the limitations of the conventional medical system.

As a seasoned developer with 30 years of professional experience, I drew on my expertise to create the tools I needed to take control of my health. Using these tools, I began my journey to **debug** my health, much like a **complex codebase**.

I created the **OpenHolter**, an open-source EKG monitor. Once EKG data capture was underway, I integrated it with a customized version of my document management platform, **Mayan EDMS**. This integration allowed me to track not just my heart but also my meals, stress levels, exercise habits, symptoms, and patterns long before the era of health apps and smartwatches.

That's when I discovered the shocking truth: my ideal diet, workouts, and supplementation were the **opposite of everything I believed, everything I'd been taught**.

I started eating animal protein, plenty of healthy fats, and almost no carbohydrates.

My workouts became focused on natural movements, neuromuscular activation, and rotation exercises.

I adjusted my supplementation with amounts that differed wildly from the daily recommended values and added things I believed were only intended for athletes.

Within months, lifelong health issues began to resolve:

- **Tachycardia**

- **Migraines**

- **Fatty liver**
- **Dermatitis**
- **Joint pain**
- **Acid reflux**
- **Insulin resistance**
- **Hypocalcemia**
- **Hypotension**
- **Brain fog**

Not only did I feel better, but the biometric data I collected and analyzed confirmed it.

This new lifestyle not only **transformed my life** but also **saved it**.

In 2025, severe abdominal pain landed me in the hospital. Doctors discovered my appendix had become **gangrenous** and **ruptured**; I should have been in **sepsis**. Instead, I went into emergency surgery with a **perfect albumin score of 5**, **no systemic infection**, a **resilient gut microbiome**, and a body primed for **rapid healing**.

In this book, I'll tell you how I did it.

I'll share the hard-won lessons from the intersection of open-source software, DIY health hardware, nutrition, and a relentless drive to figure things out for myself.

By the end of it, you'll learn how to think like a **systems engineer about your health, ask better questions**, see **hidden patterns**, and **uncover possibilities you may never have considered before**.

2

THE BUG REPORT

Diagnosing a Broken System

"No one saves us but ourselves. No one can and no one may. We ourselves must walk the path." - Buddha

Today, I'm healthier than I've ever been, even after going through emergency surgery barely **two months** ago. As I sit here finishing this book, I still find it hard to believe how far things have come. If you're reading these words, perhaps you're searching for answers too, just as I once was, and wishing for the same conclusion, minus the emergency surgery.

Not long ago, I was on a journey. It was a long, uncertain climb through self-experimentation, failures, and unexpected discoveries. I became a researcher of my biology, my own case study. I tracked everything. I built devices. At night, when my entire family was asleep, I would read medical journals until the sun came up. I questioned every assumption, especially my own.

However, to understand the intensity and the reasons behind this journey, we must go back to where it began.

Back to the first signs that something wasn't right.

My story is **shockingly unique** and yet also **paradoxically common**.

2.1   Early life

I'd had **Irritable Bowel Syndrome** (IBS) for as long as I can remember. Genetics, they said, a seemingly inescapable family history of digestive distress. My mother and her brothers battled it.

Along with IBS, diabetes is also common on my mother's side. It felt like a predetermined sentence, **a biological inevitability**.

I had to figure out which combination of foods and eating patterns triggered my symptoms, including the worst of them, sudden diarrhea, the kind that hits at the absolute worst possible moment, often in places where bathrooms were unfortunately absent.

Other times, it was intense stomach pain radiating outwards, an unrelenting ache that seemed to spread throughout my abdomen and numb my legs.

Medical examinations didn't offer conclusive answers. Appendicitis was never conclusively ruled out, nor was it ever definitively detected. Instead, I was diagnosed with chronic **right lower quadrant** (RLQ) pain, a frustratingly vague symptom with a bewildering number of potential causes, including perforated duodenal ulcers. [1]

Before the discovery that **Helicobacter pylori bacteria** cause over **90% of duodenal ulcers** and up to **80% of gastric ulcers**, stress and lifestyle factors (specifically diet and eating habits) were considered major contributors to peptic ulcer disease. [2]

Accordingly, my doctors provided dietary and eating recommendations, and that was the extent of the medical care I received for those issues.

The recommended diet, low fat, and proteins, more or less helped a bit, but it left me **perpetually undernourished**, and that led to **additional complications later on**.

Then puberty hit, and with it came abdominal bloating and acid reflux. I added antacids to the growing list of medications and remedies I carried with me everywhere.

At seventeen, I started experiencing recurring skin flare-ups that wouldn't subside. After multiple visits to dermatologists, doctors diagnosed my skin flare-ups as **Seborrheic dermatitis**. [3] I ended up with a **30-year** dependency on **Elocom** (mometasone furoate), [4] a topical steroid, to manage it.

Corticosteroids are no joke; that's why they're only available with a doctor's prescription. For me, this meant periodic visits to the doctor for refills. When they ran out, withdrawal reactions were often significantly worse and lingered far longer than the initial ailment the steroids intended to combat. [5]

At about this time, I began my martial arts journey. Being young, it was easy to stay fit, and that convinced me I had my health fully dialed in. A fortress of muscle and bone, I believed I was impervious to the usual aches and pains of aging. But my body had **other plans**.

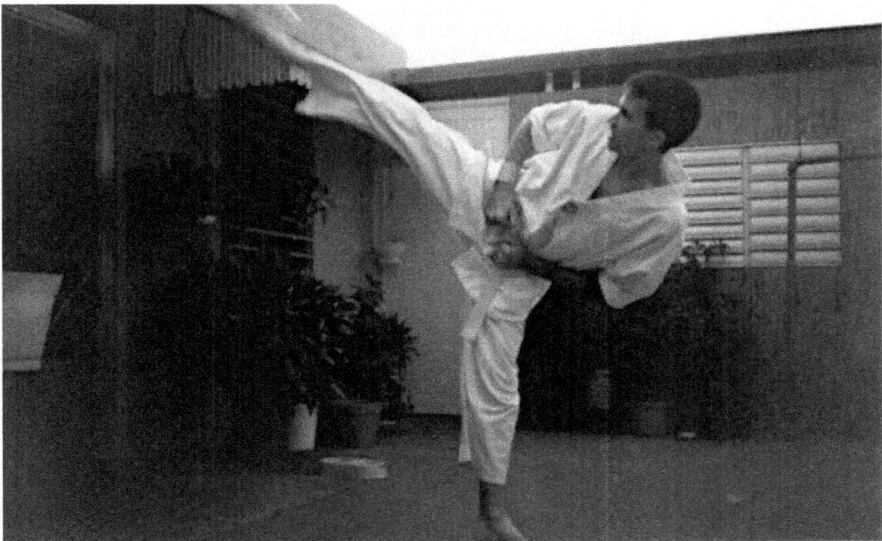

Fig. 1: Early on my martial arts journey.

2.2　Early adulthood

At twenty, persistent joint pain began to plague me. I dismissed it as stress, overtraining, a typical young adult complaint. However, taking time off and resting didn't offer any real relief.

A few years later, occasional headaches morphed into weekly migraines. I became utterly dependent on **non-steroidal anti-inflammatory drugs** (NSAIDs) just to function. These were the familiar over-the-counter painkillers, but they were **anything but docile**.

NSAIDs wreak havoc on the cardiovascular, gastrointestinal, renal, and respiratory systems, increasing the risk of gastrointestinal (GI) bleeding, causing gastrointestinal mucosal damage, oxidative damage to the intestinal mitochondria and the brush border membrane (BBM), [6] increasing intestinal permeability, [7] myocardial infarction, and stroke. [8] NSAIDs deplete glutathione, a key antioxidant and cellular defense molecule, which may contribute to oxidative stress, leading to necrosis, accelerated cell death, and potential organ dysfunction. [9]

Unknowingly, **I was compromising my most vital organs**.

*It was baffling. According to the conventional wisdom of doctors and fitness gurus, **I should have been at the peak of health**, but that wasn't the reality I was experiencing.*

The pressures of young adulthood only amplified the severity of my existing conditions. My acid reflux spiraled out of control, demanding medical attention. I cycled through doctors and endured a battery of tests, but everything came back "normal".

An esophagoscopy examination finally revealed the unmistakable sign of severe acid reflux. The doctor gave me a blunt assessment: this was essentially my fault, and also that without proactive steps, it could progress into full-blown **Gastroesophageal reflux disease** (GERD). [10]

For such a severe problem, their proposed solution was shockingly simple: avoid pizza, burgers, and other "greasy foods", don't eat after 6 PM, and take even stronger liquid antacids after dinner.

I did all that and the acid reflux intensity improved but not the frequency. The relentless backflow of stomach acid ignited chronic throat pain and recurrent throat infections, as well as laryngitis. A few months later, I began experiencing **difficulty swallowing**.

Subsequent endoscopies unveiled **oropharyngeal dysphagia**, [11] a condition that impairs the ability to swallow food and liquids. In my case, it primarily affected thin liquids, leading to frequent aspiration. Choking on water became an annoying, commonplace occurrence, and I simply learned to adapt, to swallow differently.

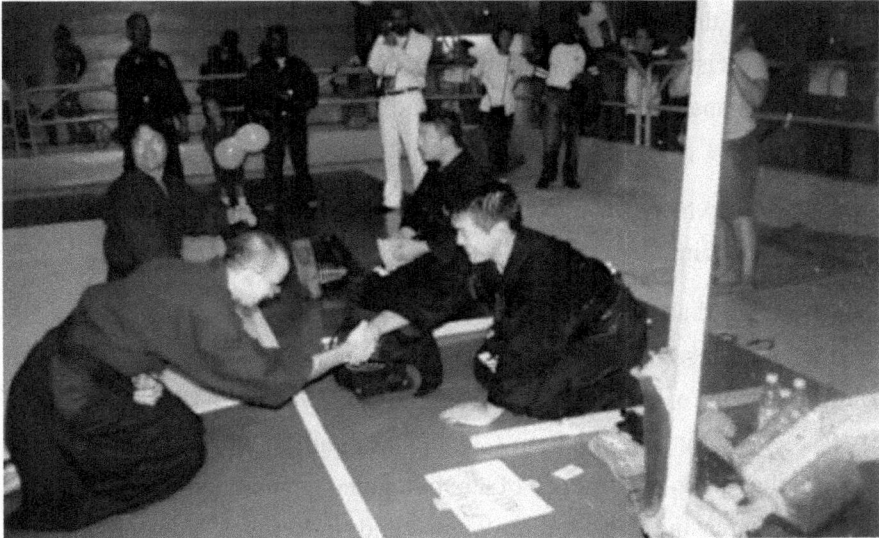

Fig. 2: Having the honor of receiving a handshake after sparing with H. Eiga, 8th dan Kendo champion and renowned master technician.

Taking more potent liquid antacids brought the acid reflux under control but made my symptoms of IBS worse. Unbeknownst to me at the time, I'd developed **Small Intestine Bacterial Overgrowth** (SIBO). The constant use of antacids had effectively reduced the acidity in my small intestine, inadvertently allowing bacteria from the large intestine to migrate and multiply. [12]

In the short term, SIBO exacerbated my IBS, but in the long term, it led to **even more complications**. [13] [14]

2.3   Later in life

In my thirties, I dove headfirst into bodybuilding, and the results were startling: I packed on a remarkable 60 pounds, swelling my 6'0" frame from 160 to 220.   This new physique undeniably boosted my self-confidence and opened doors in my social life. Yet, it came at a steep price, a **persistent fatigue** that clung to me like a shadow.

Despite the dramatic improvements in my physical appearance, my rigorous exercise routine, and meticulously planned eating habits, there was no positive impact on my underlying conditions.

It was baffling. According to the conventional wisdom of doctors and fitness gurus, **I should have been at the peak of health**, but that wasn't the reality I was experiencing.

Given my pre-diabetic history, my doctor added a liver panel as part of my routine checkups. The results identified elevated liver enzymes. The doctor told me to control my alcohol consumption. My drinking has never been excessive, and by that time in my life, it was nonexistent. He then raised the concern that given the absence of alcohol, jaundice, no upper right abdomen pain, my increasing waist circumference and **body mass index** (BMI), and high stress levels related to lifestyle and my job, the next possible diagnosis was **Nonalcoholic fatty liver disease** (NAFLD). NAFLD is the most common cause of abnormal liver test results in the United States. [15]

At forty, things went downhill; my symptoms and my conditions **all went**

into overdrive. Brain fog clung like a damp cloth, chronic fatigue was a leaden weight, and fibromyalgia pulsed with a relentless ache. Migraines became almost daily occurrences, which backed down only with a caffeinated soda accompanied by pain relievers. Dermatitis reached painful and disconcerting levels. Chest palpitations, punctuated by occasional sharp pain, intensified. I'd resigned myself to accepting these issues as simply the fallout of aging.

Annual check-ups, once a luxury, **were now a necessity**.

Despite a fasting sugar level hovering in the pre-diabetic range, a result doctors attributed to my family history, and some minor inflammation detected in my liver (dismissed as another consequence of age), everything else came back "normal".

Liver inflammation? Yes, you read that right. My liver, initially diagnosed with Nonalcoholic Fatty Liver Disease (NAFLD), had progressed to **Nonalcoholic Steatohepatitis** (NASH), a far more serious condition characterized by inflammation and damage to the liver tissue. This explained the pot belly and the persistent respiratory problems I'd been experiencing, a direct result of the inflamed liver pressing against my diaphragm.

Ironically, Nonalcoholic Fatty Liver Disease was often considered an inevitable part of life, but it was anything but harmless. Now, with Steatohepatitis, things were getting worse.

The liver plays a crucial role in numerous biological processes, [16] and **any compromise** to its function can trigger a **cascade of health problems**. [17]

Unfortunately, NASH was also exacerbating my dermatitis, rendering corticosteroids utterly ineffective. Adding home remedies like coconut oil only provided temporary relief from pain and dryness. The constant dermatitis became a continuous source of social stress.

Beyond the more aggressive dermatitis, I began experiencing a disconcerting sensation, a burning, chemical-like irritation on my upper lip. Skin irritation became increasingly common and persistently itchy, transforming into a constant, maddening issue.

To manage these escalating symptoms, I added anti-itch cream to my skincare routine alongside creams containing zinc, a standard recommendation that yielded little effect.

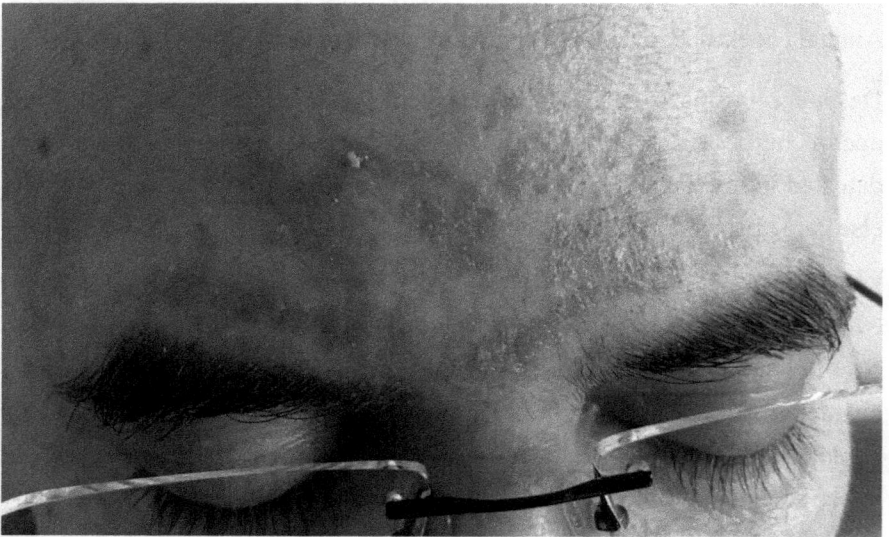

Fig. 3: Forehead dermatitis outbreak.

The recurring chest palpitations and pain prompted my doctor to order occasional EKG tests to rule out any underlying cardiac issues. Yet, these tests consistently returned "normal" results.

Still, despite these reassuring results, **I didn't feel normal. I felt profoundly broken**.

The dismissive responses from my doctors and nurses, a chorus of empty reassurances, only deepened the sense of isolation:

- *"This is all common for a man of your age"*

- *"This is nothing to worry about"*

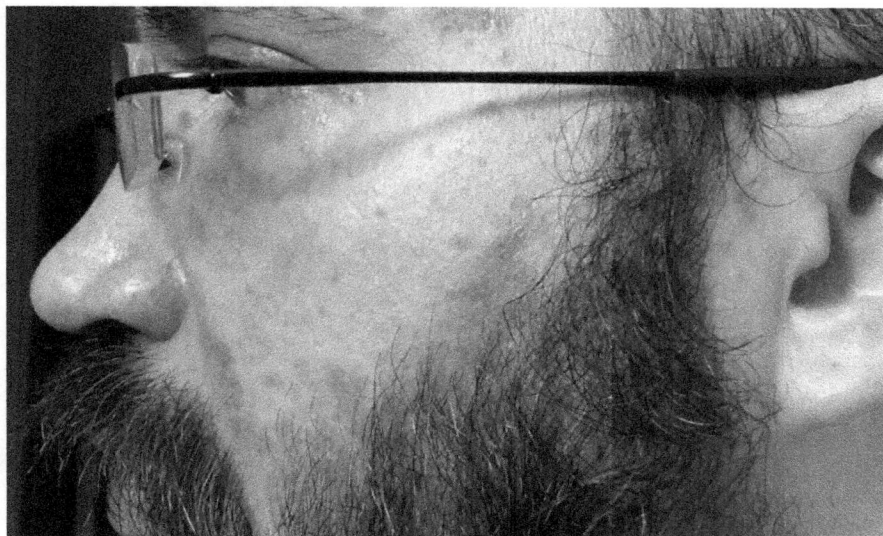

Fig. 4: Dermatitis started to cover my face.

- *"You have the blood pressure and heart rate of a teenager"*

Each phrase felt less like genuine concern and more like a polite, well-meaning deflection.

No more helpful than small talk.

2.4   The event

One night, while watching a movie with my wife, my heart suddenly began racing frantically. It was, in a sense, normal, a recurring episode I'd learned to tolerate. I relaxed, attempting to calm myself with deep breaths, holding my breath for a few seconds as I often did. This maneuver typically worked, coaxing my heart rate back to its steady rhythm. But this time, it didn't. My heart continued to speed up relentlessly.

I laid down with my legs raised in an attempt to alleviate the issue, but that didn't make a difference. Drinking plenty of water, another usual remedy, also failed to bring any relief. My heart was beating so fast and pumping so

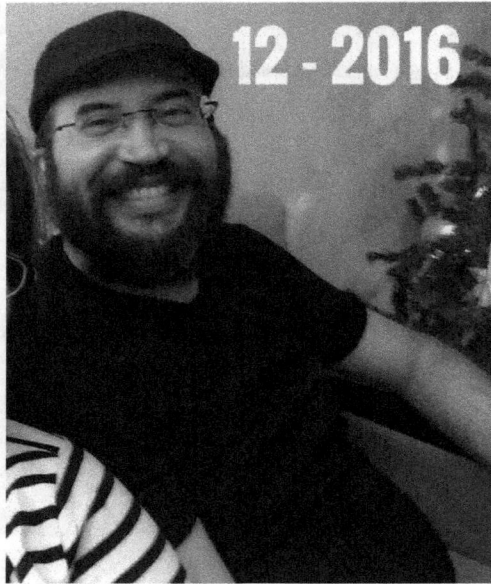

Fig. 5: My normal state in my early 40s.

hard that I could see my chest and abdomen **pounding** in rhythm with my heart.

> *As the last wisps of consciousness dissipated, I found myself lost in a morbid reverie: was this what dying felt like?*

I'm not a fan of hospitals, save for physical injuries. Therefore, I considered them and their **emergency room** (ER) a measure of last resort.

Reluctantly, I decided it was time to seek emergency medical attention. The problem was that I'd lost all strength in my body; **I was unable to stand up on my own**. With my wife's assistance, I managed to get upright, but my whole body began shaking uncontrollably.

As I stood there, my heart rate accelerated even further, causing dizziness and disorientation. My vision became blurry, and I experienced tunnel vision, the periphery of my field of view shrinking and darkening as if the world was slowly being erased around me.

With immense difficulty, my wife helped me change clothes to get ready to leave. Getting into the passenger seat demanded an almost impossible effort; I couldn't even raise my legs. Once secured, we were off on a desperate race against an unseen clock.

On the way to the ER, my wife managed to flag down police officers, who escorted us to the hospital.

As we continued, I started drifting in and out of consciousness. From that point forward, my memories fractured, becoming disjointed shards of recollection.

Upon arrival at the ER, medical staff immediately administered medication, which instantly lowered my heart rate. Relief washed over me; it seemed to resolve the immediate issue. However, as it turned out, **it wasn't quite that simple**.

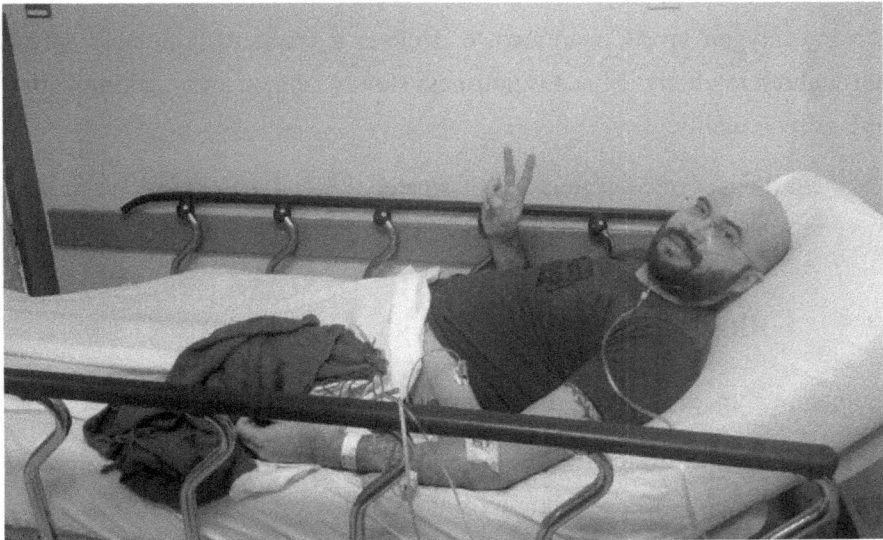

Fig. 6: The day with the worst SVT episode.

Forcefully lowering my heart rate unleashed an unforeseen consequence: my **blood pressure collapsed**, triggering a cacophony of alarms as vital signs monitors began to blare. My **oxygen saturation** levels started to drop, indicating a more serious trend.

What initially appeared to be a straightforward case of tachycardia proved to be a symptom of **something far more profound**. I was experiencing a massive **hypotension episode**. My blood pressure had dropped so low that my heart hammered frantically, attempting to compensate and push the pressure back up.

Unfortunately, when medical staff intervened, forcing my heart rate to slow without addressing the underlying hypotension, it only exacerbated the situation. The even further drop in blood pressure starved my organs, including my brain, of vital oxygen.

I plunged into a profound hypoxia, a state defined by a crippling oxygen deficiency within my body. [18] A state that, in its severity, could lead to catastrophic consequences, such as **brain damage**, **coma**, or **even death**.

As my oxygen levels continued to decline, a creeping numbness spread throughout my body. My consciousness slowly slipped away, taking with it my grip on reality.

As the last wisps of consciousness dissipated, I found myself lost in a morbid reverie: was this what dying felt like?

2.5 Follow up

Somehow, I made it. I suppose it wasn't my time.

What had been a **life-changing** experience for me was just one more case for the hospital. I was sent home from the ER with the recommendation to schedule an appointment with a cardiologist.

What followed was a slow, grinding descent into months of tests, including holter studies, stress tests, echocardiograms, and endless EKG sessions. Despite all the efforts, nothing ever pointed to a clear explanation of what was happening to me.

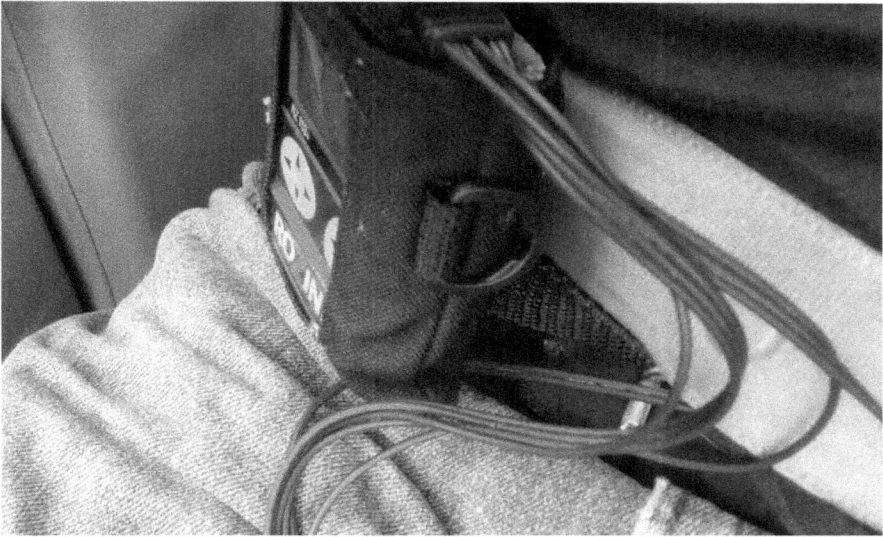

Fig. 7: One of many holter studies.

The process wasn't just slow; it was tediously prolonged, with weeks stretching between each round of testing. And then there were the administrative hurdles, surge of medical orders, insurance approvals, and the logistical nightmare of equipment leasing.

By the time I finally got the green light for the following holter study, **my symptoms had already faded**, disappearing just days before.

2.6 Diagnosis

Finally, after weeks of inconclusive tests, one holter study captured a fleeting snapshot of my episode. The following day, the hospital called, requesting I schedule an appointment.

The cardiologist delivered a diagnosis: **supraventricular tachycardia**

(SVT), causing, among other things, sustained periods of elevated heart rhythm. Not exactly a revelation, but at least it was something. I had at least a sliver of explanation.

Then came more appointments, more targeted testing, and finally, a stress test that did it. It triggered my symptoms in full again while plugged into an EKG machine. This test provoked a scenario similar to what I experienced during my ER visit. The next day, I got an urgent call from the hospital to come in for an **immediate** appointment.

This appointment went differently. The test results revealed a laundry list of heart conditions, including supraventricular tachycardia (SVT), specifically **atrial fibrillation** (AFib), **heart flutter**, **premature beats**, **low ventricular ejection fraction**, **mitral annular calcification**, mitral, tricuspid, and pulmonary **valve regurgitation**, and, most alarmingly, **nerve overgrowth**. The doctor was exceptionally emphatic that **immediate action** was necessary to address them, which felt like a dark premonition.

The heart, when functioning normally, operates like a precisely timed machine. A small cluster of cells in the sinus node initiates the rhythm, sending a single, clear signal down to the upper chambers (the atria) before flowing down to the lower chambers (the ventricles). It's a coordinated sequence, a predictable, reliable pulse.

Each beat of my heart was a brutal reminder of what I'd lost.

But in atrial fibrillation, that order dissolves. Instead of one signal, you get a chaotic burst. Multiple electrical impulses erupt simultaneously from various points in the atria, flooding the AV node and causing the heart to beat **rapidly** and **irregularly**. [19] It's like a system overload that throws the entire rhythm into disarray.

Due to this short circuit in my heart, only my ventricles were still

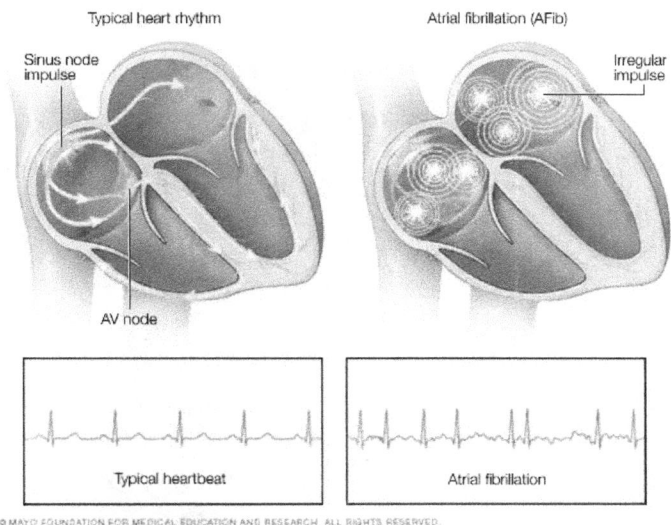

Fig. 8: Atrial fibrillation is like a short circuit in the heart's electrical system.

functioning correctly, albeit at a diminished capacity. At the same time, the atria were weakened and contracted in a disorganized manner, failing to pump blood effectively. As a result, my effective heart function was **severely compromised**.

The cardiologist recommended I undergo a heart ablation procedure to burn off the extra nerves that were causing a short circuit and restore atrial activity. [20]

My condition was so advanced that in the best-case scenario, I would need to retire by forty, stop doing sports, avoid any strenuous activities, and lead a sedentary life. In the worst case, I would need a **pacemaker** and **defibrillator**. The weight of those words settled on me, a cold, hard truth about the future I was already beginning to accept.

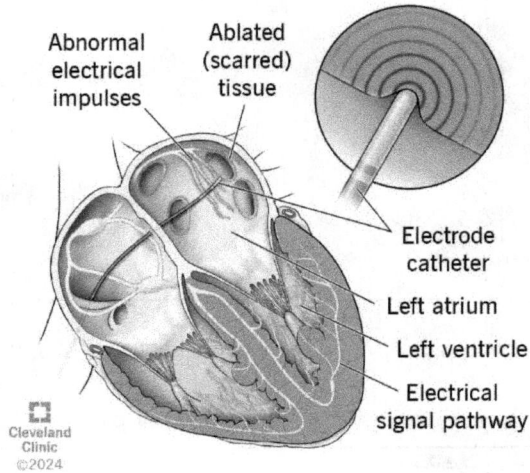

Cardiac ablation

Abnormal electrical impulses

Ablated (scarred) tissue

Electrode catheter

Left atrium

Left ventricle

Electrical signal pathway

Cleveland Clinic ©2024

Fig. 9: Cardiac ablation procedure.

2.7 Procedure

The day of the heart ablation procedure arrived. To my surprise, it was ambulatory.

I arrived very early, barely after dawn, and the staff quickly admitted me, prepped me, and then wheeled me into the operating room around 9 AM. And by 2 PM, I was being discharged. I was home before dinner.

This fix, done to my heart, felt too quick and too easy, almost like a drive-thru. How could a single, minimally invasive procedure cure so many heart issues?

Right from the very beginning, something felt **profoundly** wrong. I trusted the process and followed the post-intervention care plan and medication protocol religiously. I followed the doctors' instructions to the letter.

Yet, the rest and recovery phase came and went, and nothing changed.

The heart ablation procedure had fixed nothing. It had made things

demonstrably worse.

My tachycardia hadn't simply lingered; it had intensified, a relentless, hammering pulse that bled into every aspect of my life. The unstoppable trembling and weakness made even the simplest chores, such as walking to the mailbox or taking out the trash, feel like **monumental struggles**.

Each beat of my heart was a brutal reminder of what I'd lost.

The **only** thing that brought some relief was lying down.

I never regained my strength and my heart function after the ablation procedure. And after just a few days, my ability to do everyday things nose-dived precipitously. My energy level was barely enough to get me out of bed.

I had to adapt my gait, walking bent forward with my head level with my chest, just to maintain some semblance of normal blood pressure and heart rate. The exertion from the simplest chore left me utterly exhausted, needing constant naps throughout the day.

Those naps quickly evolved into needing to eat in bed, then progressed to eating and watching TV in bed. Eventually, I would end up having to **spend my entire day confined to bed**.

2.8   Living in my bed

The simple act of sitting up in bed, a routine that had once been utterly unremarkable, now sent a cold wave crashing through me. My blood pressure plummeted, my vision narrowed to a disconcerting tunnel, and a sickening premonition of fainting loomed. The risk of getting hurt from just leaving the bed was a depressing reality.

Suddenly, even the most basic movements and actions felt fraught with danger. I couldn't drive, couldn't even venture out for a simple stroll. I needed assistance with the most fundamental tasks of daily life, such as bathing, brushing my teeth, dressing, and even just walking to the living room.

It wasn't a gradual decline either; it was a sudden, brutal severing of my independence. My condition had rendered me **effectively disabled** and a **prisoner of my bed**.

The frustration was constant, a baffling lack of understanding surrounding my heart's erratic behavior after undergoing the procedure that was supposed to fix it.

I relentlessly pursued answers from my doctors, desperate for clarity, but the conversations were consistently unproductive, almost **dismissive**. They weren't overtly hostile, not precisely, but there was a palpable distance, a disconcerting disconnection, a feeling that they were simply **uninterested in delving deeper**.

My persistent pleas for answers, which they seemed incapable of providing, invariably triggered a perceptible irritation, or worse, a rapid-fire deluge of excessive technical jargon and obscure medical terms to justify my current state.

The end of each consultation always felt like a calculated maneuver, a thinly veiled suggestion that **I was the problem** in the situation. That I must simply accept the scenario as "typical", be patient with the process, endure, and follow their indications. And always, methodically, the reminder that if things did not improve, the solution was a pacemaker and defibrillator, my **Sword of Damocles**.

This wasn't medical advice; it felt like improvisations cobbled together on the spot, lacking any real foundation in research or genuine concern. The result was a profound sense of confusion and alienation, a feeling of being utterly adrift in a system that **refused to acknowledge my humanity**.

I began to stare at my short-term future, a bleak landscape of unemployment, reliance on others, a life confined to a bed, and a crushing **burden on my**

family. The thought of being unable to care for my family, **not being able to even care for myself**, was a suffocating realization. Even with my wife taking on more cases at work, the bank account was dwindling and drying up.

Desperate, with no viable options remaining, the path forward became clear: If I wanted to uncover the truth about my health, I needed to **take matters into my own hands**. At this point, **I didn't have much to lose**.

3

BUILDING THE OPENHOLTER

Hardware as a Health Mirror

"The impediment to action advances action. What stands in the way becomes the way." - Marcus Aurelius

My goal wasn't to create a medical device. It was a desperate attempt to silence the suffocating feeling that I was **slowly dying**.

Despite its endless rounds of retesting the same things, the medical system could only provide the same reassuring platitudes, nothing but an unhelpful *"You're doing just fine"*. But my **agonizing body** was telling a **different story**.

Beyond the increasingly concerning heart issues, a persistent undercurrent of suffering remained.

They were the old skin problems, a source of almost constant pain all over my face and my scalp and spreading into my upper back and chest.

The relentless acid reflux that burned its way up my throat, forcing me to sleep either in an almost sitting position, propped up with three pillows, or on my left side. Any other position jolted me awake with a sharp pain in my already burned and swollen esophagus and throat.

The pain in my bones and joints was a constant, unwelcome guest. I managed to dial it down only with painkillers and by rubbing vaporizing pain remedies that gave me temporary, deceptive relief.

The debilitating fatigue that clung to me like a shroud. Even with sleep medication that allowed me to get eight hours of sleep, I would still wake up feeling as if I'd settled for a fraction of that.

And then there was the tangled mess of gut issues that seemed determined to sabotage my every attempt at normalcy.

These weren't abstract symptoms; they were a **daily, brutal reality**.

3.1 Everything starts with a necessity

Frustrated by the complete absence of answers and the feeling that I was being systematically ignored, I turned to the only thing I truly trusted: data. Not the carefully curated, sanitized data presented in a doctor's office but raw, unvarnished information.

Consumer-accessible medical monitors were an emerging market, still in its early stages, and faced significant challenges in gaining traction. They were scarce, severely limited, and prohibitively expensive. For an unemployed patient adrift in a sea of uncertainty, they were simply **beyond reach**.

Even today, with the breathtaking advancements in processing power, miniaturization, and sensor technology, most devices offer only the barest of metrics: steps taken, hours slept, and heart rate, often with a not insignificant margin of error. These metrics, while superficially pleasant, were inadequate for my needs. They were like glancing at a weather report and assuming you understood the entire season.

What I desperately needed was something far more profound: **raw, real-time, high-resolution** data on what my heart was doing, not just during brief clinic visits or fleeting snapshots captured in a controlled environment. I needed a deeper, more nuanced understanding of my physiological responses to the myriad stimuli.

The technology simply hadn't caught up. It hadn't learned to listen to the language of my body.

3.2 Perseverance

Despite being bedridden, I still possessed a lifeline: **the internet**, accessible through my phone, and a **mind stubbornly refusing to surrender**.

Lying in bed, I devoured everything I could find on heart tachycardia, arrhythmia, and the labyrinthine world of cardiac pathologies. Managing the symptoms wasn't enough; I needed to know what was happening within the confines of my body.

We ordered a copy of my medical file, a request that seemed to register with the doctors as a deliberate act of aggression. Their behavior suggested they viewed my inquiry as a hostile challenge, a prelude to **questioning their decisions** in a legal battle.

The file itself was a collection of fragments: lab results, EKG readings, prescriptions, clinical notes, and the standard, sterile documentation of a patient's illness.

However, as I consumed it, a sense of disappointment settled over me. The reports felt disconnected, like pieces of a puzzle scattered across a vast, empty room. Each data point provided a limited, isolated view, devoid of context, of the larger system. **There was no continuity**.

It was data, yes, but data that had already yielded its predictable fruit, offering no new insights and no potential for additional or alternative treatments. It was, for lack of a better term, "hospital data", a recorded set of observations, useless beyond the walls of the institution, divorced from my lived experiences or my current reality.

Years of working on information technology taught me the type of challenge I was facing: I was diagnosing a **black box**, a system whose internal workings remained opaque, its behavior determined solely by its inputs and outputs.

I had the only two things I needed: ***motivation*** *and* ***information***.

Ironically, the very advances in technology that had propelled us forward, the relentless pursuit of speed, efficiency, and complexity, had simultaneously rendered the art of diagnosis a lost one. We'd become so adept at building intricate systems, layers upon layers of code and circuits, without truly understanding what lay beneath. We optimize for performance, for metrics, and for the illusion of control, often without considering the consequences.

Now, we're **drowning in our creations** while simultaneously experiencing a creeping erosion of our **ability to understand them**. It's a dangerous trend, a slow forgetting of the fundamental principles that once grounded our ability comprehend complex systems.

My experience with this pattern in the world of technology helped me realize that a similar phenomenon was occurring in medicine and our approach to health. The reductionist model, which treats symptoms in isolation and categorizes conditions as if they were independent errors, reflects the same flawed mindset.

So, I began to approach the problem differently. Instead of seeing my health as discrete conditions neatly categorized and treated in isolated silos, I started to understand it as a complex, interconnected system responding to thousands of interwoven influences.

This shift in perspective was crucial. It would allow me to perceive the intricate web of interactions, the subtle feedback loops, and the way my body responded not just to the artificial, controlled environment of the hospital but to the natural rhythms and influences of my environment.

That intent required a perspective beyond the confines of a single examination room or a single set of test results. It demanded a willingness to delve into the data, to seek the patterns hidden beneath the surface.

I needed to build a model, **a living, breathing model of my health**, that encompassed everything and, crucially, related it to the environment surrounding me.

Diagnosing the symptoms alone wasn't enough; I needed to understand the underlying architecture of my being. To understand it and open myself up to new and **innovative solutions**, as well as **possibly even treatments**.

3.3   Necessity leads to ideas

I realized I needed data from my production, a lot of it, to understand the fundamental mechanisms driving my condition.

So, I did what any developer would do: I decided to **build my own diagnostic tool**.

My first step was researching how a holter monitor worked. Essentially, it's an EKG with a time component, creating a histogram of the heart's electrical activity over a specified period. Basically, they are data loggers.

Thanks to my previous experience in manufacturing, I had valuable experience using, diagnosing, and building data loggers, as well as programming PLCs and microcontrollers.

I had the only two things I needed: **motivation** and **information**. I could build a simple holter monitor for my purposes.

Since my condition had confined me to bed for most of the day, I would absorb as much information as I could. Then, I would draft plans to execute at night during the one hour I would spend moving around to get a minimal amount of exercise. I had set up my work area and got started.

It didn't take long before I had a proof-of-concept up and running. It was gratifying to see my heart wave displayed on a small screen held in my hand.

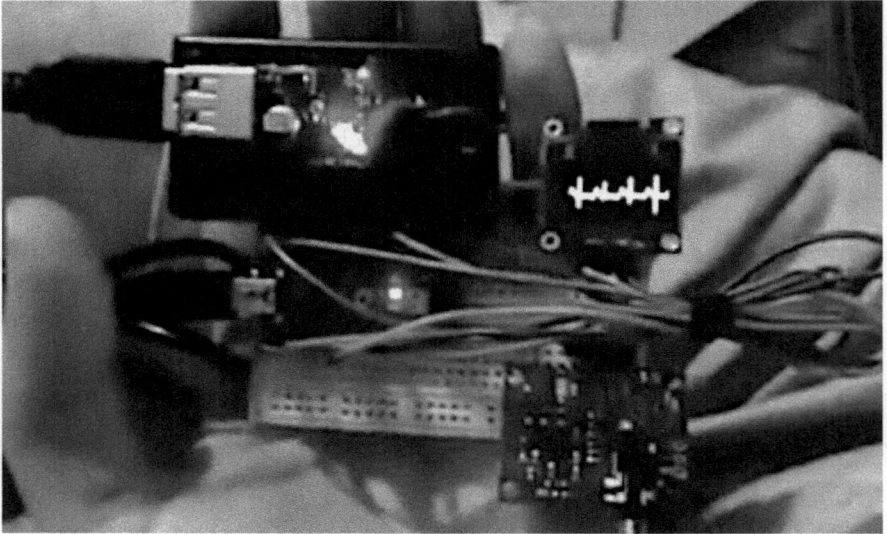

Fig. 1: OpenHolter proof of concept.

Over the next few days, I refined my design and created a prototype that was compact enough to carry around on a protoboard. This portable prototype helped me prove the project's actual viability.

It was a success!

I could see how my heart reacted to stress as I got out of bed and how it behaved when I lay down.

Motivated by these results, I designed the third iteration. This one would be housed in an enclosure and feature a user interface, a self-contained power supply, and improved firmware.

After a few nights of work, it was complete. **I had created the OpenHolter.**
21 22

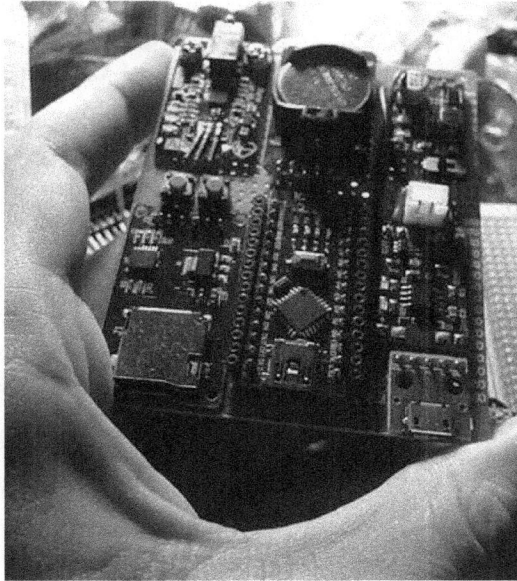

Fig. 2: First OpenHolter prototype.

3.4 Design

At its core, the OpenHolter is a **do-it-yourself (DIY), wearable, open-source EKG holter device**, a continuous heart monitoring system that captures and records the heart's electrical activity.

Unlike clinical holter monitors, it's affordable, transparent, and built with off-the-shelf components that anyone can source. It can also be expanded, improved, and modified.

Total cost of **$30 US dollars**. **No hidden firmware**. **No locked-down ecosystem**. Only pure, raw heart data, on my terms.

3.4.1 Processor

The foundation of the OpenHolter's hardware design lies in a remarkable microcontroller board: the **Arduino Nano**.

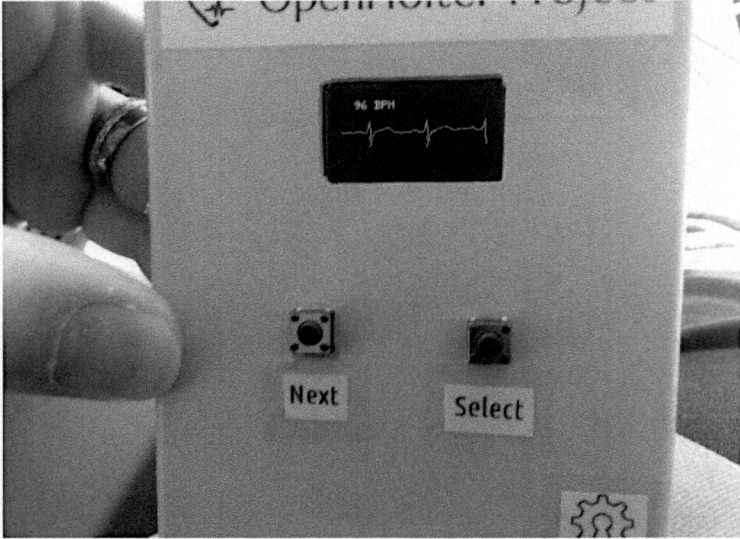

Fig. 3: First fully model of the OpenHolter.

This compact, versatile, and affordable microcontroller board is built upon the well-documented and thoroughly understood **ATmega328P chip**. [23] [24] The Arduino Nano shares similarities with its larger counterpart, the Arduino Uno, but boasts a more portable form factor, making it ideal for applications where space is limited.

The Arduino Nano operates at a frequency of **16 MHz**, which, by today's standards, might appear insufficient. However, the Arduino Nano, unlike a computer, does not run an **operating system** (OS). This means that the microprocessor runs only one program, allowing developers to tap into the full capabilities of the microcontroller unhindered by the overhead of an OS.

It supports digital communication protocols such as **Inter-Integrated Circuit** (I^2C) and **Serial Peripheral Interface** (SPI). [25] [26] These protocols are essential for fast and efficient communication in embedded systems, offering several advantages over traditional binary parallel or serial communication methods.

For instance, I^2C and SPI enable lower cable counts, reducing the complexity

Microcontroller unit - Arduino Nano

- Clones at $4 USD
- Atmel Atmega 328 at 16 MHz
- Analog and digital pins
- 32 KB Flash (minus 2KB bootloader)
- I2C & SPI communications
- UART TTL to USB

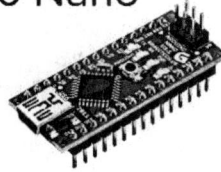

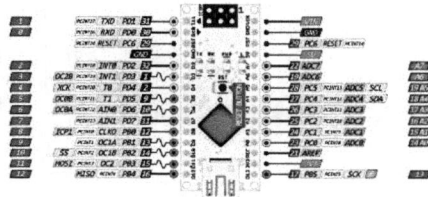

Fig. 4: Arduino Nano.

of system design and improving device addressing. While I^2C and SPI may have lower bandwidth compared to raw serial or parallel communications, their benefits far outweigh the costs in the context of the OpenHolter project.

Besides supporting digital protocols, the Arduino Nano features an integrated **analog-to-digital converter** (ADC), enabling the conversion of real-world signals into digital data.

The Arduino Nano's architecture provides **32 KB of flash memory** for storing code, **2 KB of RAM** for runtime values, and **1 KB of non-volatile EEPROM** for storing settings and other content that needs to persist between power cycles.

The Arduino project's original goal was to create an accessible, low-cost platform for non-engineers, yet it has proven itself capable of powering more complex applications. [27] [28]

The successful integration of the Arduino Nano in the OpenHolter project is a testament to its **versatility and power**.

Block diagram - Communications

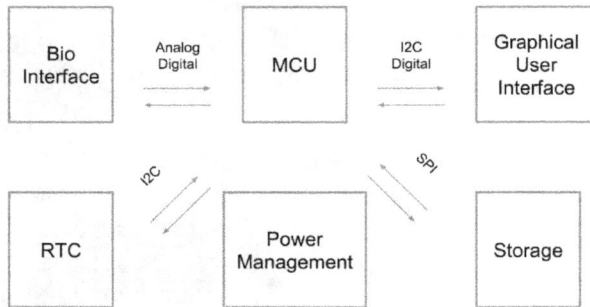

Fig. 5: Block diagram - communications.

3.4.2   ECG Frontend

The next crucial component for the OpenHolter is the biological interface, a link that enables the device to capture the subtle biopotential signals emanating from the human body. However, the ADC built into the Arduino Nano was not sufficient for this task. The ADC's limitations necessitated the addition of a specialized analog-to-digital frontend specifically designed to acquire and process biopotential signals.

After searching for self-contained modules that could meet these requirements, I narrowed down my options to the **AD8232 ECG module**. [29] This analog front end is engineered to extract and amplify millivolt-level electrical signals generated by cardiac activity.

I chose the AD8232 for several compelling reasons. Firstly, it struck an optimal balance between features, price, power consumption, and form factor. Secondly, besides the basic functionality expected of a frontend module, it boasts a range of innovative features that make it an ideal choice for biopotential signal acquisition:

- **Leads-off detection**: This feature prevents the device from recording

Bio Interface - Analog Devices AD8232

- $10-$20 USD
- Built-in voltage comparators
- Built-in amplifier
- Built-in filtering
- Power management
- Cons: No ADC

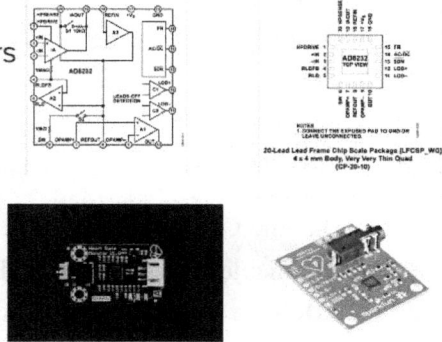

Fig. 6: AD8232 ECG frontend module.

blank or erroneous data, akin to taking photos with the camera cap still in place.

- **Integrated reference buffer**: The AD8232 generates a virtual ground, which is essential for maintaining signal integrity and reducing noise.

- **Support for multiple electrode configurations**: The module can accommodate either two- or three-electrode setups, offering greater flexibility and adaptability.

- **Multiple operation modes**: It can capture ECG waveforms in both stationary and portable settings, with the added benefit of motion artifact elimination, a crucial feature for ensuring accurate signal readings while wearing the holter.

- **RFI filtering**: Designed to operate in noisy environments, the AD8232 includes internal **Radio Frequency Interference** (RFI) filters that help minimize **electromagnetic interference** (EMI).

- **Fast restore feature**: This feature enables quick recovery from abrupt signal changes.

- **Electrostatic discharge (ESD) protection**: The module's **Human Body Model** (HBM) rating of 8 kilovolts provides good ESD immunity, safeguarding against damage caused by electrical discharges.

3.4.3 Real-time clock

To ensure that the OpenHolter accurately timestamped the ECG recordings, it required a reliable **real-time clock** (RTC) on board. For this component, I chose the **Dallas DS3231**, a well-documented integrated circuit (IC) that's widely used in the industry. [30]

Real Time Clock - Dallas DS3231

- $1 USD
- I2C Interface
- Unlike DS1302 and DS1307, has temperature compensated crystal and crystal oscillator
- Has battery input and powerless timekeeping

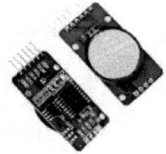

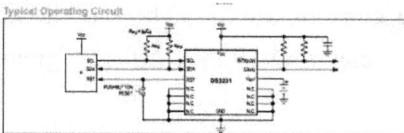

Typical Operating Circuit

SQUARE-WAVE OUTPUT FREQUENCY

RS2	RS1	SQUARE-WAVE OUTPUT FREQUENCY
0	0	1Hz
0	1	1.024kHz
1	0	4.096kHz
1	1	8.192kHz

Fig. 7: Real time clock used, the Dallas DS3231.

It supports I^2C communication for seamless compatibility with the Arduino Nano, eliminating the need to implement custom device communication protocols.

Many popular modules for the DS3231 IC also support the installation of a coin cell battery. Adding a battery to the RTC enabled the OpenHolter to maintain accurate timekeeping even when it's powered off, thereby reducing the likelihood of assigning the incorrect date or time to ECG recordings.

The DS3231 features a built-in **temperature-compensated crystal oscillator** (TCXO), which automatically adjusts in response to temperature changes. This feature ensures that the timekeeping system remains incredibly precise, even in environments with fluctuating temperatures.

But precision isn't the only advantage of this IC; it also includes a **square wave generator**, a vital component for **real-time software applications**.

3.4.4 User interface

When designing the OpenHolter, my primary goal was to utilize it throughout the entire day under various lighting conditions. This goal meant that display readability was very important.

After experimenting with different LCD models, I ultimately chose **Organic Light-Emitting Diode** (OLED) technology. Although hobbyist OLED displays were scarce and pricey in 2016, their exceptional resolution and contrast ratio are hard to beat.

Another key advantage of OLED technology is that it's self-illuminating, removing the need for backlights that can be prone to damage by physical shock. Using an OLED display also allowed for faster refresh rates compared to LCDs, a crucial aspect for correctly visualizing the ECG waves.

Following extensive research and supplier scouting, I selected the **Solomon Systech OLED display model SD1306**. [31] Although it falls on the lower end of the cost spectrum, this display model supports I^2C communication, a fast refresh rate, and very low image retention.

To handle user input, I implemented a basic setup of two push buttons to minimize cost and complexity.

Each button functions in multiple modes:

Graphical User Interface - Solomon Systech SD1306

- $5 USD
- Multiple communication modes including I2C
- OLED
- Visibility
- Pixel based
- 2 x Push buttons

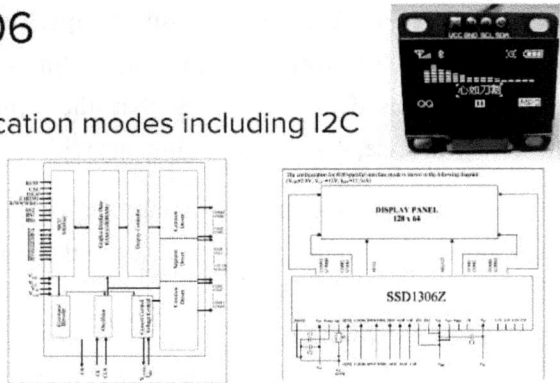

Fig. 8: User interface is accomplished using the OLED display model SD1306.

- Next and Select

- Ok and Cancel

For driving the display and capturing user input, I used the **U8g2 library**. [32] This library supports an extensive range of display models, font rendering, graphic drawing, and high-level features such as graphical user interface (GUI) components, handling physical buttons, and button debouncing.

Button debouncing is a technique used to prevent multiple unwanted signals from being registered when a button is pressed, particularly in mechanical switches. This feature significantly increased the reliability of the user interface without requiring me to write custom debouncing code.

3.4.5 Accuracy

To capture the ECG signal with high precision, the OpenHolter's software had to be designed from the ground up as a **real-time system**. To meet this critical requirement, I employed **interrupt-driven programming** techniques.

Interrupts are a mechanism that allows a device or a program to signal to the CPU that it needs to handle an event, causing the CPU to temporarily suspend its current execution and jump to a specific section of the code. This code section is referred to as the **Interrupt Service Routine** (ISR).

This is where the DS3231's square wave generator comes into play. By connecting the square wave generator's output to the Arduino, I could trigger precise interrupts that would perform biosignal sampling.

Sampling rate reliability - Solution

Use the DS3231 square wave output pin to trigger Arduino's hardware interrupt and do sampling in an ISR.

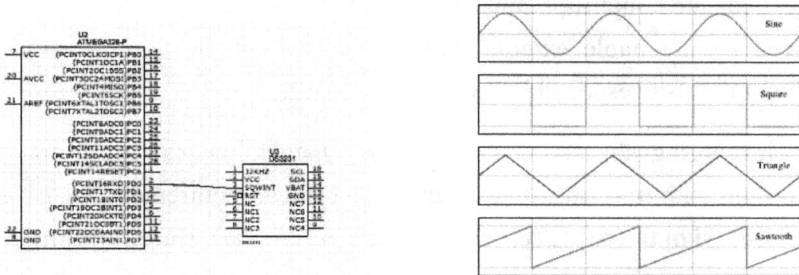

Fig. 9: The output square wave generator of the DS3231 is used as an interrupt signal source for the Arduino.

When it comes to triggering interrupts, the Arduino Nano offers two main options: **Pin Change Interrupts** (PCINTs) and **dedicated external interrupt pins**.

PCINTs have several limitations that make them less suitable for the OpenHolter's design.

For one, PCINTs divide pins into groups, with all members of a group sharing a single interrupt line. This means that any pin state change within a group triggers the same interrupt and executes the same ISR. The ISR code must then run an additional check to determine which specific pin caused the interrupt, a process that adds unnecessary complexity.

Furthermore, PCINTs can only be triggered by a change in pin state.

In contrast, dedicated external interrupt pins offer individualized interrupt lines for each pin, which allows for individual ISR calls without additional code. These pins also allow for more flexibility in terms of trigger modes, including rising edge, falling edge, or change events.

The Arduino Nano's pins **2** and **3** are wired directly to the internal hardware interrupt lines, **INT0** and **INT1**, providing a reliable foundation for the ECG measurement process.

The dedicated interrupt pins' ability to deliver individualized interrupts, driven by a reliable external timer, makes them the optimal choice for driving the ISR responsible for ECG sampling.

By leveraging this combination, the OpenHolter can perform signal sampling with **deterministic intervals**, a critical requirement for achieving **precise signal capture resolution**, **accurate timestamping**, and **downstream temporal analysis** such as **heartbeat detection**, **RR interval calculation**, and **heart rate variability (HRV) determination**.

Despite being a homemade system, this design aspect of the OpenHolter is the primary characteristic that **propels the project beyond the hobbyist scope** and into the more serious medical device landscape.

3.4.6   Cables

The OpenHolter's electrode setup utilizes the three leads system: **right arm** (RA), **left arm** (LA), and **right leg** (RL). This configuration ensures good signal quality while rejecting common-mode noise.

Initially, I made my own cables, but this method proved time-consuming and inadvertently introduced unwanted noise into the samples. As the project progressed, I explored commercial cable brands to identify more suitable alternatives.

Organic interface - Connectors

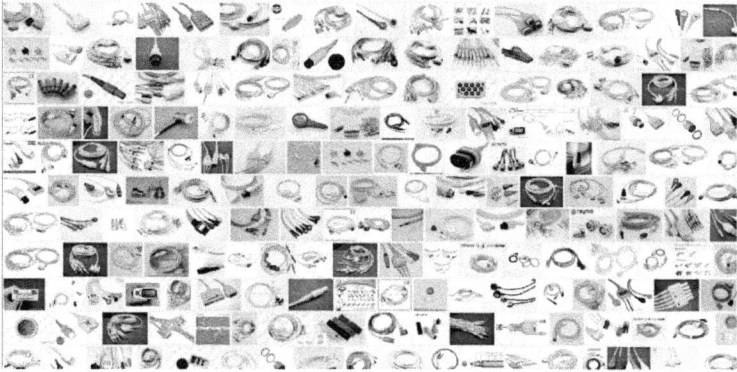

Fig. 10: Large variation of ECG electrode cables.

However, this approach presented its own set of challenges: cables are often designed with proprietary machine connectors that cater to specific ECG machine brands, limiting compatibility and versatility.

The vast array of available cables necessitated an exhaustive research process, which included multiple purchases, trial-and-error interface testing, and evaluation of each cable's characteristics.

When selecting the ideal cable for the OpenHolter application, I considered several criteria: **clip connector quality**, **wire gauge**, **tangle resistance**, **total length**, and **clear connector labeling**.

The quest for a suitable cable was far from straightforward, as many retail options lacked branding or explicit product information. As such, visual inspections became the primary means of evaluation, resulting in multiple purchases before I could identify the optimal cable.

Organic interface - Leads

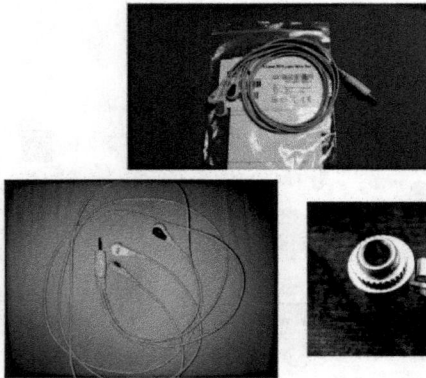

- Professional ones
  - Best connectors
  - Best wire gauge
  - Tangle resistant
  - Labeled
  - $20 USD
  - Easy to interface

Fig. 11: Researching ECG electrode cables.

One obstacle in developing the OpenHolter's interface arose when attempting to acquire the corresponding machine connectors for the cables, an almost impossible task due to their proprietary nature.

Nevertheless, a moderate selection of cables featured mechanically and electrically compatible connectors that mirrored those found on **audio equipment**. Seizing this opportunity, I sourced different audio jack connectors and repurposed them as cable-machine interfaces, effectively bypassing the challenge posed by proprietary connectors.

The realm of ECG cables and connectors presents a notable opportunity for standardization, which would significantly enhance interoperability, mitigate obsolescence, and reduce costs.

Open standards, or even industry standards beyond the current **ANSI/AAMI EC53**, [33] [34] would advance the professional and hobbyist medical communities' ability to develop new equipment and conduct innovative experiments in cardiometry, such as the OpenHolter.

3.4.7 Electrodes

The process of selecting the right electrodes was similar to choosing the right cables, extensive and requiring trial and error until narrowing down the options to several viable brand models.

Organic interface - Electrodes

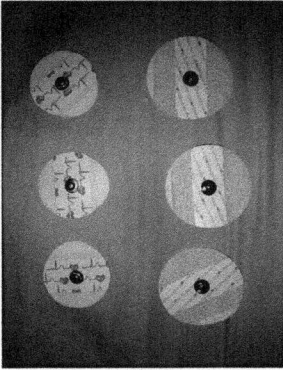

- BIO Protech T815
  - Cloth
  - Extended wear (day)
  - Sweat resistant
  - Cons: Painful to remove
- BIO Protech T716
  - Foam
  - Cons: Not water resistant

Fig. 12: Researching ECG electrode types.

One notable exception stood out: **Bio Protech**.

Their model **T716** proved to be a suitable choice for experimentation as well as casual use.

However, for extended periods of usage, I found the model **T815** to be an excellent option. This cloth-based electrode model offers exceptional breathability and resistance to sweat.

3.4.8 Power management

I designed the OpenHolter primarily as a portable device. To that end, I also added an on-board power supply.

At its core lies a single-cell **lithium-ion (Li-ion) rechargeable battery**, [35] which provides approximately **12** days of continuous recording. This battery technology boasts a superior power density compared to alkaline batteries.

Even in 2016, lithium-ion batteries were widely available and abundant, making them a good choice for the OpenHolter. Moreover, besides buying them brand new, lithium-ion cells can be repurposed from damaged laptop batteries and other consumer products, reducing electronic waste. Even used Li-ion batteries can still provide sufficient power to sustain the OpenHolter's operation for multiple days.

A voltage inverter module is employed to boost the battery's **3.7** volts to the **5** volts required by the Arduino and the components. A secondary power management module handles recharging the lithium-ion battery.

Power management - Custom

- GTL 18650 5300mAh Lithium Ion ($2 USD)
- Lithium Ion charger module w/ output pins ($0.35 USD)
- 3.7v to 5v voltage inverter ($0.50 USD)

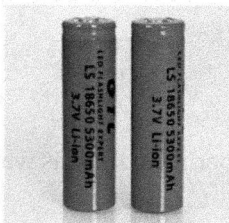

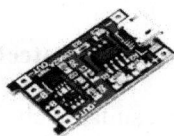

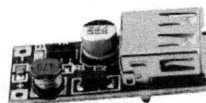

Fig. 13: Power management solution centered around lithium-ion battery technology.

Power consumption is meticulously managed at the firmware level, leveraging the Arduino's sleep modes during idle cycles to minimize energy draw.

A dedicated external USB port provides a centralized interface for easy access. By connecting the Arduino's USB port and the charging module to the external USB port, the OpenHolter can handle **firmware uploads**, **serial communication**, and **charging operations** through a single USB cable.

3.4.9 Storage

After my experience with the limitations of holter studies, for the OpenHolter, I wanted a **high-capacity**, **non-volatile** media so I could store more ECG recordings and not worry about losing them if the device lost power.

As with the other components, ease of use and price were important selection criteria. **Secure Digital** (SD) flash memory cards, although proprietary, are very common, cost-effective, and easy to interface. I opted for the **microSD** form factor to conserve space.

Since writing to the SD card is slower than capturing the ECG samples, the samples are stored in a memory buffer and then written to the card in bulk. This method mitigates wear on the SD card and optimizes writing throughput.

This usage of an SD card achieves the design goals:

- The OpenHolter can sustain **extended recording sessions**, exceeding the capacity of many commercial devices.

- Stored ECG recordings are **safe** even when the OpenHolter loses power.

- The recordings can be **easily downloaded** from the OpenHolter via the USB cable or by physically ejecting the SD card and inserting it into an SD card reader.

- Communication with the SD card was **simple**, achieved using the SPI protocol.

For seamless integration with the SD card, the firmware uses **Bill Greiman's SDfatlib library**. [36]

Storage - SDCard & module

- $3 USD (card) + $1 USD (reader)
- Cons: Fast modes need license.
- SPI bus mode. This bus type supports only a 3.3-volt interface. This is the only bus type that does not require a host license.
- 5V to 3V converter
- 5V to 3V level converter

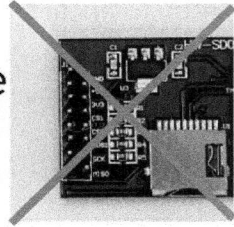

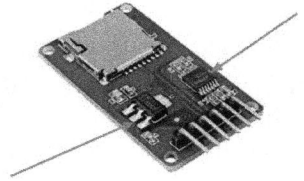

Fig. 14: MicroSD cards are used for long-term storage of ECG data.

For simplicity and compatibility, the OpenHolter stores the digitized ECG data in **Comma-Separated Values** (CSV) format. Each line represents a timestamped sample, where the time is measured in milliseconds since the recording commenced, followed by the ECG frontend output as captured by the Arduino's ADC.

The CSV format offers several advantages, including **easy parsing**, **analysis**, and **portability**. To facilitate future-proofing and backward compatibility, a header is added to each file, indicating its version number. If new ECG recording formats are implemented, the software loading the recording can quickly identify the correct version, utilize the proper format specifications, and read the file content correctly.

The Arduino Nano's 2 KB SRAM constraint necessitated careful consideration of using **static buffers** and avoiding **slower dynamic memory allocation**. To address this challenge, a **circular buffer** is implemented to manage data storage efficiently. This approach allows the ISR to push data into the buffer and rapidly return, minimizing its runtime

Recordings format

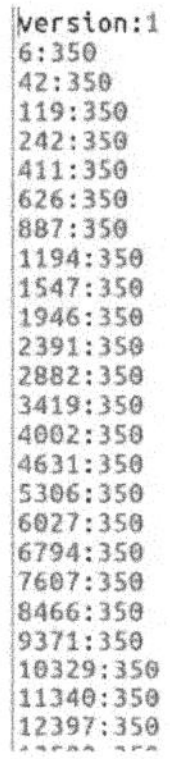

```
Version:1
6:350
42:350
119:350
242:350
411:350
626:350
887:350
1194:350
1547:350
1946:350
2391:350
2882:350
3419:350
4002:350
4631:350
5306:350
6027:350
6794:350
7607:350
8466:350
9371:350
10329:350
11340:350
12397:350
```

Fig. 15: The file format used to store ECG values.

while ensuring uninterrupted operation. In parallel, the main loop reads the buffer and writes to the SD card at its own pace.

To conserve memory further, I did not use all the features of the SDfatlib library. The SD card is formatted in **FAT32**, but **FAT16** ASCII filenames are used, avoiding the need for Unicode support.

Given that recordings use a time offset, it's essential to encode the start time and date within the filename of each recording CSV file. However, FAT16 files are limited to 8.3 filenames (eight characters for the name and three characters for the extension). With the fixed "CSV" extension, this leaves only eight characters to encode the date and time.

To overcome this constraint, the recording's start date and time get converted to **Unix time**. This system represents timestamps as the number of seconds that have elapsed since the **Unix epoch** (January 1, 1970, at midnight UTC). This numerical representation facilitates easy storage, comparison, and calculation with dates and times. The resulting Unix time is then converted to hexadecimal format, yielding an 8-digit hexadecimal number.

Recordings format

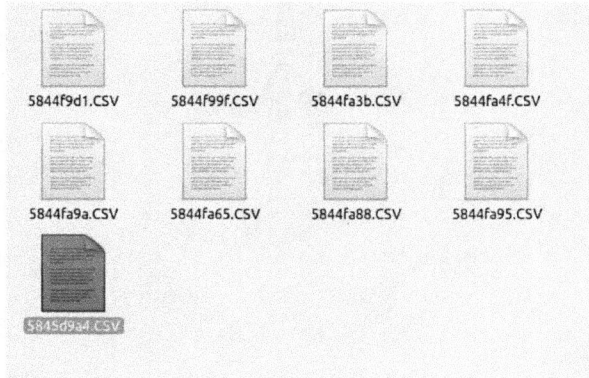

Fig. 16: Filename scheme used for ECG recordings.

For instance, **February 1, 2017, 11:00 PM GMT** corresponds to Unix time **1485946800**. When converted to hexadecimal, this becomes **5891BFB0**. This approach offers a straightforward yet robust solution for encoding dates and times within filenames.

Moreover, this method offers an ample range of dates beyond the maximum expected lifespan of the project, with a maximum date that can be encoded corresponding to **February 7, 2106 (0xFFFFFFFF)**.

3.4.10   Modes

Initially, the OpenHolter functioned solely in standard holter mode, where ECG measurements were recorded to the SD card without any additional features or interactions. However, its open platform design facilitated firmware updates, enabling the addition of more modes of operation.

One such update introduced a real-time ECG display mode, enabling the monitoring of heart activity similar to that of a traditional EKG machine. In this mode, the OpenHolter displays a real-time ECG wave, accompanied by a heart rate counter and heartbeat indicator. This mode is excellent for obtaining immediate feedback on how various activities, exercises, or posture changes affect the cardiovascular system in real time.

A subsequent update introduced an ECG transmission mode. This mode configures the OpenHolter to capture ECG data and transmit it to a computer connected via its USB port. In this configuration, the OpenHolter, in conjunction with a computer, transforms into an EKG machine capable of advanced functionalities, such as:

- **ECG wave freezing**: pause and examine specific segments of the heart rhythm

- **ECG wave comparison**: analyze and contrast different recordings for diagnostic purposes

- **Real-time ECG wave analysis**: leverage the processing power of the computer to perform complex analyses that would be impractical or impossible with the Arduino Nano microcontroller alone

3.5   The first breakthrough

With the third iteration model completed and in use, I could immediately see the changes in my heart rate and ECG waveform as my heart stress increased when I changed posture or performed basic activities.

It was during this experimentation that the term **"posture"** caught my attention. In my research, I've read about **Orthostatic hypotension**, also known as **postural hypotension**.

Orthostatic hypotension (OH) is a medical condition characterized by a sudden drop in blood pressure when standing up from a sitting or lying down position. It occurs because the body's autonomic nervous system fails to compensate adequately for the decrease in venous return and cardiac output that happens when assuming an upright posture. [37]

I also learned about **Initial Orthostatic Hypotension** (IOH), which equally causes Postural Tachycardia. However, this effect is only transient and considered normal. [38]

I found that the symptomatology of OH was a very close fit to my own experiences and observations.

To test the hypothesis that OH might be related to my heart issues, my wife got compression socks, specifically, the type used by long-distance runners. To my surprise, with the compression socks on, the stress on my heart diminished when sitting up, and I could see this reflected in the live heart wave on my OpenHolter.

I had my Eureka moment!

This realization was a turning point for me: I wasn't just dealing with an isolated issue; I was looking at a **cascade failure**.

In computer science, a cascading failure occurs when a malfunction in one part of a system triggers a chain reaction, resulting in failures in other interconnected components. As the chain reaction continues, the original malfunction eventually spreads to components that **might not seem connected** to the origin of the problem. This **domino effect** can occur in complex systems such as computer networks, large software projects, power grids, distributed systems, or, in my case, my own body.

In my case, I observed and validated that my heart tachycardia was not an isolated issue but rather a symptom of a cascading failure in my cardiovascular system. There was a vascular issue triggering a chain reaction, causing sustained episodes of hypotension, and this led my heart to overcompensate by beating faster and harder.

Things began to make more and more sense. My heart **was not** the source of the problem. It was **reacting** and **picking up the slack** for something else. Not just now but for most of my entire life.

The **lifelong overcompensation** had been causing **low-grade chronic**

myocardial infarctions.

That's why my blood tests consistently showed the presence of **Troponin**, which becomes elevated in acute myocardial infarctions but, in my case, was always at **subclinical levels**. [39] [40] [41] [42] That was also the reason the electrocardiograms never found anything. They were **only** looking for telltale signs of acute myocardial infarction, such as **Q waves** or **ST-segment elevation**, which I didn't have. [43]

Unlike an **ST-segment elevation myocardial infarction** (STEMI), **non-ST elevation myocardial infarction** (NSTEMI) doesn't show a specific, recognizable change in the heart's electrical activity on an electrocardiogram. While NSTEMI causes less immediate harm than a STEMI, it still compromises the **heart's oxygen supply**, resulting in ongoing, **progressive damage**. [44] [45]

Following each myocardial infarction, the **nerve growth factor** (NGF) level increases, in turn promoting **sympathetic nerve sprouting** in the heart. While this may be part of a regenerative response, it can also lead to **heterogeneous reinnervation**, in which the nerves reconnect to a mixture of muscle fibers not initially targeted by the nerve. This disruption of electrical signaling and muscle activation increases the risk of **malignant arrhythmias**. [46]

This insight was both enlightening and chilling. If I did not solve the underlying problem that was causing my tachycardia, the nerve growth factor would cause my **heart conditions to relapse**. I would end up in a **worse position** than I was in when all of this started.

I had the next piece of the puzzle. But what caused the hypotension in the first place?

3.6   A plan takes shape

As I continued to use the OpenHolter, I began recording EKG data from various activities, including sleeping, eating, working, and exercising, at every second and every beat. As a software developer, I knew exactly what to do next: look for patterns and correlations.

However, having the hardware and the raw data without insight is akin to noise. The OpenHolter was an excellent starting point, great for collecting data, but I needed more. I required activity data and a way to make sense of the readings. I needed a **long-term electronic health journal** where I could enter, store, and analyze many data points from several sources.

Then it clicked: I already had just the thing. That's when **Mayan EDMS** came into play.

4

CONNECTING THE DOTS

Mayan EDMS as My Health Journal

"Whatever you do, work at it with all your heart, as working for the Lord, not for human masters," - Colossians 3:23

The phrase "correlation does not imply causation" resonated deeply with me as I worked with the data streaming from my OpenHolter. Data like a torrent of heartbeats, subtle fluctuations, and hidden irregularities, all of which were captured in real-time. Now, I needed causation.

A spike in heart activity? Okay, interesting. But what triggered it?

A dip in heart rate variability? Sure, that's noted. But was it stress, a heavy meal, or simply fatigue?

It became clear: the heart data was **just one piece** of a vastly more complex puzzle. The fundamental insights wouldn't come from simply observing the data; they'd require connecting it to the underlying causes.

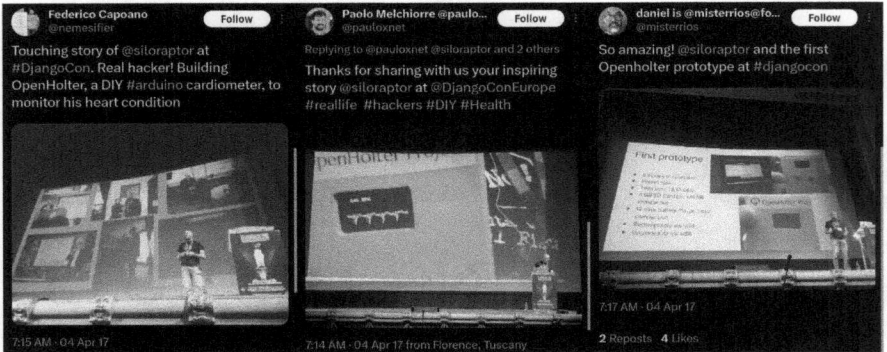

Fig. 1: Tweets about the OpenHolter presentation at DjangoCon Europe, 2017.

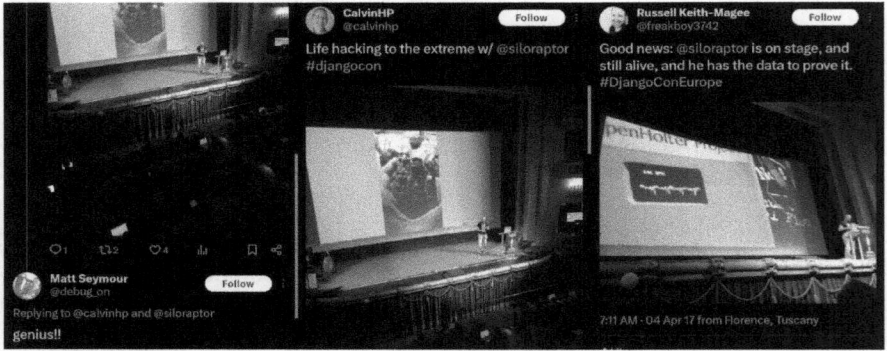

Fig. 2: Tweets about the OpenHolter presentation at DjangoCon Europe, 2017.

4.1 Adding software

Beyond the heart data, I realized I needed a way to capture a comprehensive picture of my life, a holistic view that could reveal the **connections**.

To achieve this goal, I turned to a tool I'd already built: **Mayan EDMS**.

Mayan EDMS is a powerful document management system designed for enterprise environments, such as law firms, research institutions, governments, and large organizations that require structured access to documents on a large scale. [47] [48]

But now, its purpose has shifted dramatically. It was no longer about managing legal briefs or government records; it was about my life.

So, I transformed Mayan EDMS into something entirely new: **a precision health journal**.

Short term findings were very interesting but what really blew my mind was the long term analysis.

4.2   Design

I built a custom app for Mayan EDMS, specifically designed to process OpenHolter EKG data.

This custom solution allowed me to import ECG recordings and render them using an interactive histogram control, providing quick access to every section of the data.

Crucially, the app also enabled me to link each recording to a wealth of contextual information, transforming raw data into **actionable intelligence**.

4.2.1   The foundation

I built Mayan EDMS upon **Django**, a **Python** framework for web apps.

However, what sets Mayan EDMS apart is its superset nature; it's not just a document management system but also a development platform. It expands on Django by incorporating additional reusable features, such as user interface widgets, forms, navigation, permissions, and more.

To kick start the app-building process, I leveraged **Cookiecutter Django**, a framework for creating Django projects quickly. [49] I forked Cookiecutter Django and extended it to develop Mayan EDMS apps. [50]

Once the starter app is created, it needs to be made accessible. This is accomplished by creating a single link definition and binding that link to the tools menu.

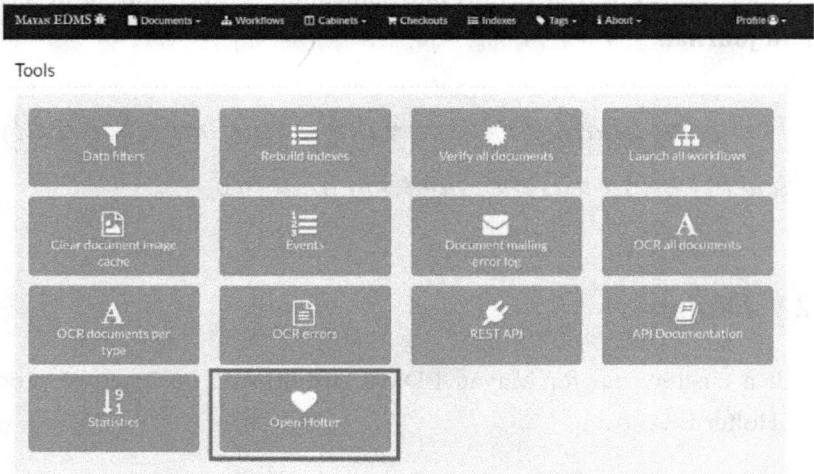

Fig. 3: The OpenHolter app is registered in the Mayan EDMS tools menu.

4.2.2 Models

To store the uploaded ECG recordings, I defined two models within the app. One model tracked the CSV files (*Recordings*), while the other stored the ECG values and their corresponding time dimension (*RecordingData*).

```python
class Recording(models.Model):
    datetime = models.DateTimeField(
        blank=True, unique=True, verbose_name=_('Date time')
    )
    file_field = models.FileField(
        upload_to=UUID_FUNCTION, verbose_name=_('File')
    )
    ready = models.BooleanField(default=False, verbose_name=_(
↪'Ready?'))

    class Meta:
```

(continues on next page)

(continued from previous page)

```python
        verbose_name = _('Recording')
        verbose_name_plural = _('Recordings')

    def __str__(self):
        return force_text(formats.localize(self.datetime, use_
↪l10n=True))
```

```python
class RecordingData(models.Model):
    recording = models.ForeignKey(
        Recording, related_name='data', verbose_name=_('Recording')
    )
    datetime = models.DateTimeField(db_index=True, verbose_name=_(
↪'Date time'))
    value = models.IntegerField(verbose_name=_('Value'))

    class Meta:
        ordering = ('datetime',)
        verbose_name = _('Recording data')
        verbose_name_plural = _('Recordings data')
```

Adhering to Django's philosophy of "fat models", which encourages developers to centralize application logic within the model layer, I added a *Recording* class method named *.process()* to handle the processing of ECG recordings.

```python
def process(self):
    self.data.all().delete()

    with self.file_field as file_object:
        # Magic number
        data = file_object.readline()

        if data != OPENHOLTER_FILE_MAGIC:
            raise OpenHolterInvalidRecordingError(
                'Invalid magic number; {}'.format(data)
            )
```

(continues on next page)

(continued from previous page)

```
        # Version
        data = file_object.readline()
        if data != OPENHOLTER_VERSION:
            raise OpenHolterInvalidRecordingError('Invalid version␣
↪number')

        data = file_object.readline()
        while(data):
            timestamp, value = data.split(':')
            date_time = self.datetime + datetime.
↪timedelta(milliseconds=int(timestamp))
            self.data.create(datetime=date_time, value=int(value))
            data = file_object.readline()

    self.ready = True
    self.save()
```

4.2.3   Views

Thanks to Mayan EDMS's reusable and extensible view classes, adding screens for uploading, deleting, viewing, and listing recordings required minimal code.

```
class RecordingCreateView(SingleObjectCreateView):
    fields = ('file_field',)
    model = Recording

    def get_extra_context(self):
        return {
            'title': _('Upload a new recording')
        }



class RecordingDeleteView(SingleObjectDeleteView):
    model = Recording
```

(continues on next page)

(continued from previous page)

```python
    def get_extra_context(self):
        return {
            'title': _('Delete recording: %s?') % self.get_object()
        }


class RecordingDetailView(MultiFormView):
    form_classes = {
        'comments': RecordingCommentForm,
        'document_type': DocumentTypeSelectForm,
        'recording_preview': RecordingPreviewForm,
        'tags': TagMultipleSelectionForm
    }
    prefixes = {
        'comments': 'comments',
        'document_type': 'document_type',
        'recording_preview': 'recording',
        'tags': 'tags'
    }
    template_name = 'appearance/generic_form.html'


class RecordingListView(SingleObjectListView):
    model = Recording

    def get_extra_context(self):
        return {
            'hide_link': True,
            'title': _('Recordings list')
        }


class RecordingProcessView(ConfirmView):
    def get_extra_context(self):
        return {
            'hide_link': True,
            'title': _('Process recording: %s?') % self.get_object()
        }
```

(continues on next page)

(continued from previous page)

```
def get_object(self):
    return get_object_or_404(Recording, pk=self.kwargs['pk'])

def view_action(self):
    task_process_recording.apply_async(
        kwargs={
            'recording_id': self.get_object().pk
        }
    )
```

4.2.4   Data entry

With the base views completed, I turned my attention to creating a data entry system.

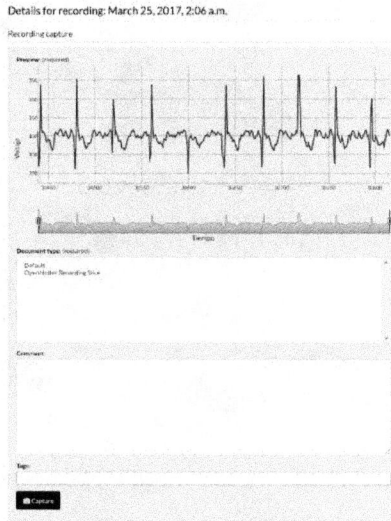

Fig. 4: Mayan EDMS app form to capture holter recordings. Note: the ECG wave is inverted on the Y-axis. This is an artifact of the analog-to-digital conversion, which was later addressed, along with amplitude adjustments and wave denoising.

I crafted a custom form to display a preview of the ECG values and included an interactive control for examining the recording. I also leveraged this interactive control to allow uploading the entire recording or a specific fragment.

4.2.5 Indexing

Once I uploaded the recordings into Mayan EDMS, I could treat them like any other document, leveraging all the platform's features.

As the number of recordings grew, it became essential to classify and index them. Mayan EDMS excels at this task by providing **automated indexing** and **classification** features. [51] To organize the recordings, I created a simple two-component index that partitioned recordings by year and month.

Tree template nodes for index: Creation date

Total: 3

Level	Enabled	Has document links?			
Root	✓	✗	New child node		
↳{{ document.date_added|date:"Y" }}	✓	✗	New child node	Edit	Delete
↳{{ document.date_added|date:"m" }}	✓	✓	New child node	Edit	Delete

Fig. 5: Creating an index template to categorize recordings.

Later on, I added more complex indexing strategies, such as partitioning by **symptoms**, **time of day**, and specific **keywords** from the recording comments.

Mayan EDMS's indexing system is dynamic and fully automated. Once the

Contents for index: Creation date / 2017 / 03

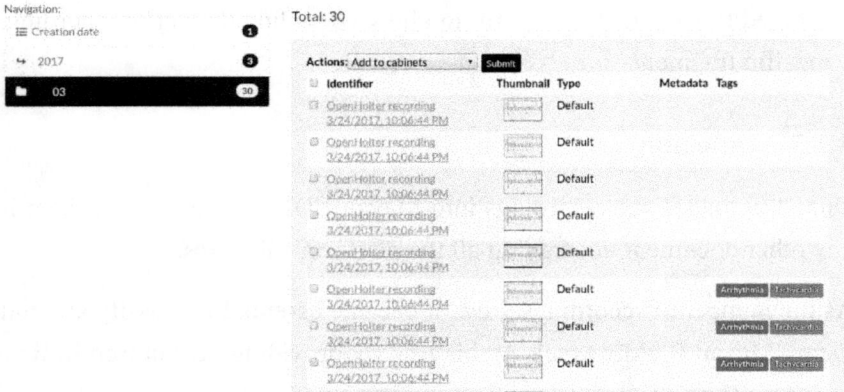

Fig. 6: Navigating a populated index template of recordings.

index is defined, recordings are automatically classified when they are created, edited, or deleted. With this configuration in place, I could focus on uploading as many recordings as possible without worrying about the organization. Later, I could build a new taxonomic structure using a fresh index template and instantly all recordings through an entirely different layout.

4.2.6   Search

Having the ability to search recordings also became a crucial aspect of this system.

Mayan EDMS supports full-text searching, allowing me to use any attribute as search criteria. Recordings could be searched by comments, dates, or tags.

With the app completed, I started uploading recordings constantly and adding crucial details like:

- **What I ate** (notes, macronutrient breakdowns)

Dashboard

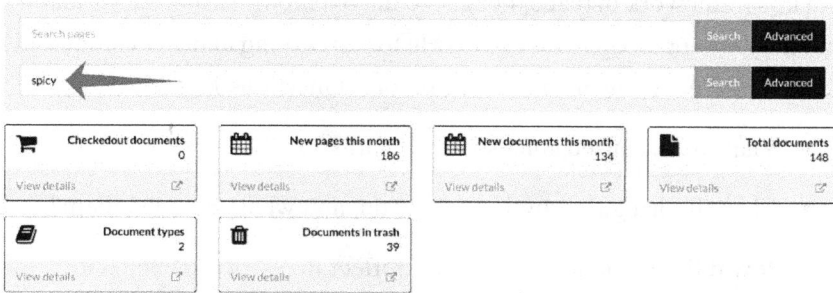

Fig. 7: The main search bar can be used to find recordings by any attribute.

- **How I slept** (hours, interruptions)

- **Physical activity** (type, duration, intensity)

- **Stressful events** (source, type, duration, aftermath)

- **Symptoms** (acid reflux, brain fog, IBS)

Since Mayan EDMS is a comprehensive document management system, I also uploaded **photos of my food**, **condiments**, and **food nutrition labels**, as well as related **research papers** and scanned copies of my **lab results** and **test reports**.

I then used Mayan EDMS's smart links feature to reference each of these documents to specific recordings, creating a thorough web of interconnected information. I was making a **mind map of my health**.

Suddenly, my life felt less like a chaotic stream of consciousness and more like an easily **searchable codebase**. This system allowed me to look for correlations and to consider rigorously the potential links between my choices and my heart's response. It was like debugging a complex program, only instead of fixing code, I was **troubleshooting** my biology.

With this framework in place, I began to uncover long-term insights that were genuinely eye-opening. I was now able to start asking and answering critical questions I'd never even considered before. Questions like:

- What foods caused spikes in my heart stress?

- When did irregular rhythms show up, and what preceded them?

- How did my gut and liver issues reflect in my heart's behavior?

I now had the tools and correlated information to **debug my health**.

4.3   Grinding halt

Thanks to the new Mayan EDMS app and the **actionable correlations** it provided, my health was turning a critical corner. At last, after a long time, I was well enough to drive and work. The fog that had hung over my days was lifting, my energy was returning, and progress felt undeniably real.

But then things took a dramatic, almost cinematic turn.

Puerto Rico got hit by a hurricane. Not just a storm. A **catastrophe**.

Hurricane Maria slammed into the island with a ferocity that defied description; in a howling wind and torrential rain, the world we knew vanished. [52]

You never truly appreciate how dependent modern life is on invisible systems until those systems disappear. Flip a switch, and nothing happens. Turn on the tap, and you're met with an unsettling silence. Cell phones turn into inert slabs of glass and metal. Your computer becomes an expensive paperweight.

It wasn't just discomfort; it was a profound disconnection. A creeping isolation as everything you took for granted begins to collapse. And the hurricane, as devastating as it was, was only the prologue. The real disaster was just starting.

4.3.1 Aftermath

Hours blurred into days. Days stretched into weeks. One month later, there was still no power, no clean water, no telecommunications, and no medical care. The island was adrift, cut off from the world.

The government's response? **A monumental failure**. [53]

The full scale of the failure wouldn't come to light for years. But for us living through it, we didn't need an official report to tell us what we already knew: **help wasn't coming**.

Many lives were lost, some during the storm, the immediate toll, but many more in the weeks that followed as a consequence of the living conditions forced upon us.

Some drowned, others starved, and others still died of dehydration, untreated illness, or the ultimate despair that settles in when hope vanishes. [54]

The official death toll? **2,975**. [55] Some estimates put it as high as **4,645**. [56]

The OpenHolter had already proved crucial to my health. Now, with no access to hospitals, clinics, or even phone consultations, it would become essential to my survival.

4.3.2 The scenario

In the pitch-black nights of the post-hurricane blackout, the design choices of the OpenHolter **shone again**.

Its OLED screen was perfectly readable in the complete darkness. The lithium-ion battery gave me nearly two weeks of use per charge. I could still take ECG recordings and also perform spot diagnosis.

But there was a new problem. The SD card design allowed the OpenHolter to hold numerous recordings, but without power, I could no longer use my desktop computer to download the ECG logs or journal my symptoms. I was **one square back**.

Journaling also became more critical than ever as new variables entered the equation. Variables that would challenge even the healthiest person, let alone a recovering heart patient.

- The constant **stress** of surviving without the basic necessities.

- The **anxiety** of not knowing if family members were alive.

- The physical toll of performing **heavy tasks** by hand, like washing bedsheets and hauling water. Things that technology had long since automated.

- The unstoppable deterioration of our emergency **food supply**. The lack of fresh food forced us to survive on our emergency stash of canned goods. As those also ran out, we were left with emergency food loaded with carbohydrates and heavy preservatives, a diet **designed for survival, not health**.

I had to get my health journal online again. Fast.

4.3.3   Energy crisis

Puerto Rico is an island that imports **85%** of its food, fuel, and medicine. [57] With all ports of entry closed those national supplies were dwindling rapidly.

In the first few days, we used our car to charge the OpenHolter and other essential devices. As the blackout stretched on, earning the grim label "America's Biggest Blackout", [58] the gas in our car quickly became a **precious commodity**, something to be guarded and not wasted.

Our condominium complex forbade power generators. Even if they had been allowed, given the circumstances, and if I could obtain one by chance, there was no infrastructure in place to interconnect them with the building's

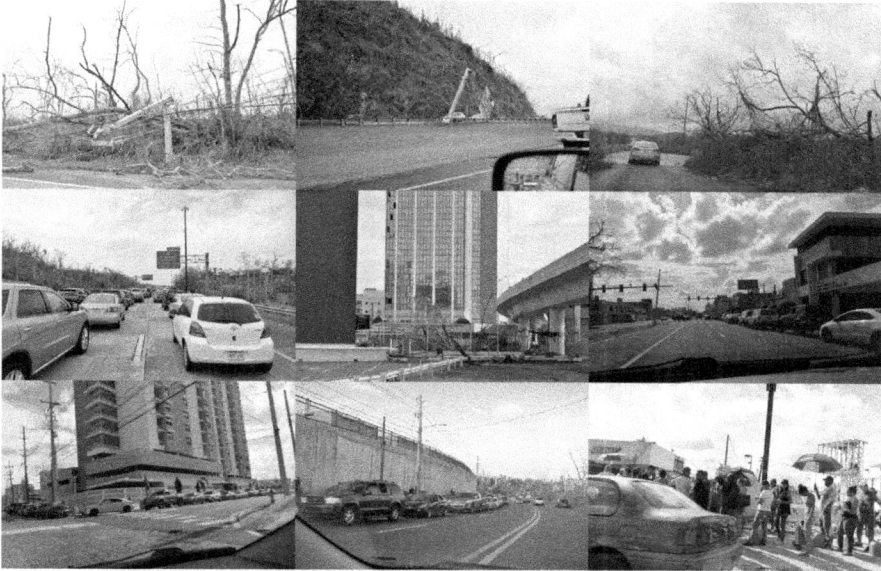

Fig. 8: Photos of the aftermath of Hurricane Maria.

electrical systems safely. Not that it mattered much, as gas was practically **unobtainable**.

Debris clogged the roads for weeks. When the government and volunteers finally cleared the roads from debris, the gas stations were either closed or buried under **miles-long** lines of cars and people on foot. Gas rationing was quickly imposed. You could wait for hours only to be told you were allowed a minimal amount. These frustrations immediately led to social unrest and even worse consequences. The government was forced to post police personnel on gas stations. Desperation gripped the island, and it was **best to stay indoors**.

I had plenty of emergency water left, and the emergency food, although not healthy, would still last for a considerable time. However, it was clear that the problem with gas would not be solved soon; energy would not be available for a **long time**.

Once again, circumstances were against my health recovery. And so, once again, I took matters into my own hands and engineered another solution.

4.3.4 Carving a path

Hardware stores were closed, and the postal system was still down. If I wanted something, anything, I was going to have to build it **myself** with **whatever** I already had around.

It took me a day to make an inventory and brainstorm. Soon after, I had a plan and a bill of materials:

- One old 75-watt solar panel

- A used deep-cycle battery

- An old **Uninterruptible Power Supply** (UPS)

- DC-DC converters, the kind used for remote-controlled drones

- Several Odroid **single-board computers** (SBCs)

- A few older but functional laptops

- Spare parts left from OpenHolter experiments

And with that, the **solar-powered microserver farm** was born.

Yes, it was part hacker project, part survival gear. But it worked. MacGyver would've nodded in approval.

The idea was straightforward: to create a compact, off-grid solar power system. Then, power the single-board computers (SBCs) using the DC-DC converters and use the UPS as an inverter to charge the laptops that would serve as workstations.

And it worked. [59]

These were not just simple devices; they were packed with purpose. I leveraged existing open-source software stacks to provide them with features typically reserved for much larger setups, such as remote serial console access for out-of-band system management. [60]

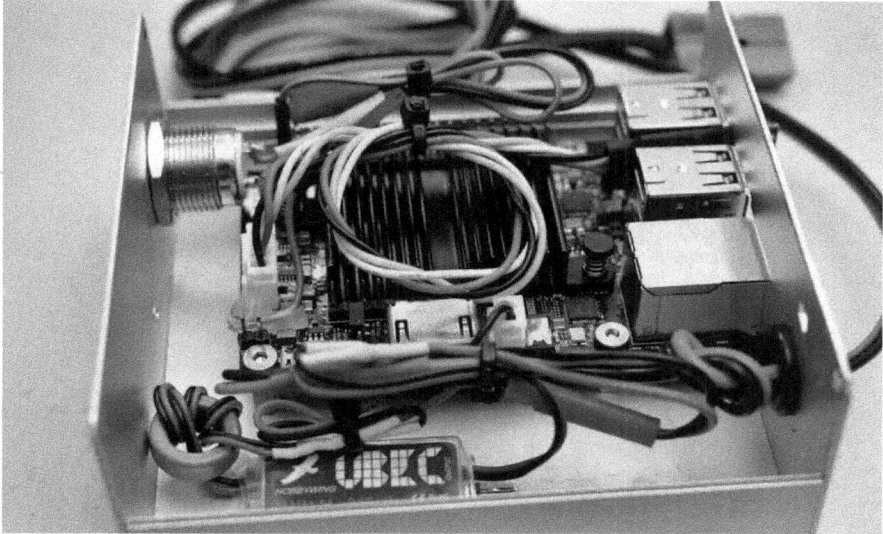

Fig. 9: Solar-powered microserver in an aluminum enclosure with wireless remote management.

I set up some of the devices as a **network-attached storage** (NAS). [61] Using a **distributed filesystem**, I had a unified storage layer across multiple servers. [62] This allowed me to use my storage devices as a single logical unit, providing efficient storage and retrieval of data while also increasing data redundancy and failure tolerance.

I configured other devices as compute nodes, designated only to run programs. I had Mayan EDMS installed and running on these. [63] Health journaling was back online. My OpenHolter data was safe.

When the world started to crawl back toward normalcy, I didn't wait. I invested in higher-capacity deep-cycle batteries, additional solar panels, a proper charge controller, and a heavy-duty inverter. I had a fully operational, **solar-powered, off-grid home lab** that was resilient and ready.

This system helped me continue earning an income, develop critical software, and, most importantly, improve my health.

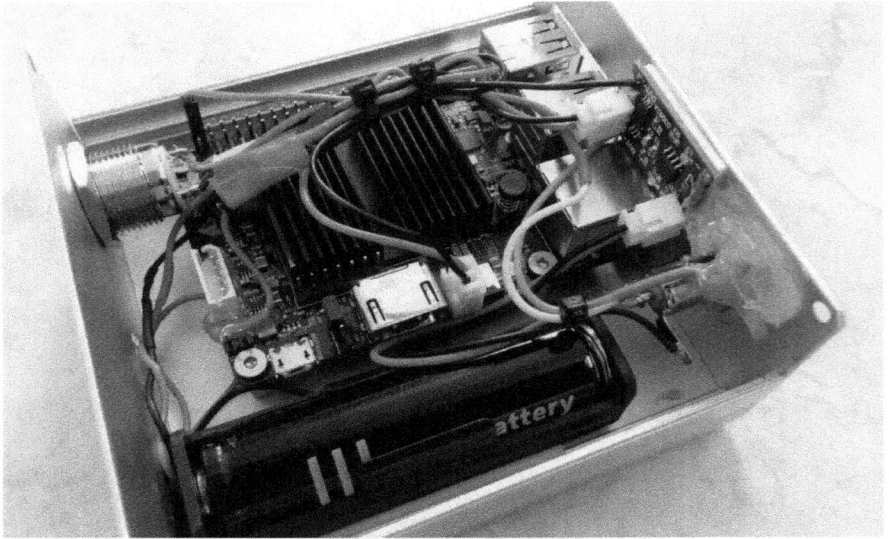

Fig. 10: Another variation of the solar-powered microserver, this one with an 18650 lithium-ion battery and charger. These microservers had their own built-in mini UPS.

And the island's health? It was still in the early stages and barely recovering.

But my journey? My path to wellness had resumed and was at **full speed**.

4.4　Things start to make sense

The short-term findings were exciting, but what truly blew my mind was the long-term analysis.

While activities and stressors did impact my heart readings, the most significant factor was not what I had expected. The most **crucial** factor was **food**. It was unmistakable: certain foods consistently triggered abnormal heart rhythms and blood pressure issues.

My body had been sending me signals all along, but I hadn't been paying attention. I had become conditioned to ignore them. The OpenHolter didn't just record data; it gave me the **power to listen**, **analyze**, and **understand**

All documents

Total (1 - 40 out of 147) (Page 1 of 4)

Actions: Add to cabinets ▾ Submit

	Identifier	Thumbnail	Type	Metadata	Tags
☐	OpenHolter recording 3/24/2017, 10:06:44 PM		OpenHolter Recording Slice		Arrhythmia
☐	OpenHolter recording 3/24/2017, 10:06:44 PM		OpenHolter Recording Slice		
☐	OpenHolter recording 3/24/2017, 10:06:44 PM		OpenHolter Recording Slice		Arrhythmia Tachycardia
☐	OpenHolter recording 3/24/2017, 10:06:44 PM		OpenHolter Recording Slice		Tachycardia
☐	OpenHolter recording 3/24/2017, 10:06:44 PM		OpenHolter Recording Slice		Arrhythmia Tachycardia
☐	OpenHolter recording 3/24/2017, 9:26:26 PM		OpenHolter Recording Slice		Arrhythmia Tachycardia
☐	OpenHolter recording 3/24/2017, 10:06:44 PM		OpenHolter Recording Slice		Arrhythmia Tachycardia
☐	OpenHolter recording 3/24/2017, 10:06:44 PM		OpenHolter Recording Slice		Arrhythmia
☐	OpenHolter recording 3/24/2017, 10:06:44 PM		OpenHolter Recording Slice		Arrhythmia
☐	OpenHolter recording 3/24/2017, 10:06:44 PM		OpenHolter Recording Slice		
☐	OpenHolter recording 3/24/2017, 10:06:44 PM		OpenHolter Recording Slice		

Fig. 11: Mayan EDMS app view showing a list of tagged recordings.

my body in a way that was previously inaccessible to me.

The OpenHolter, in conjunction with Mayan EDMS, became more than a device and software; they became a **mirror**, one that reflected to me how my daily inputs shaped my internal reality. Unlike a wearable that gamifies steps or calories, this system respects the complexity of the human body. It didn't try to simplify, filter, or dumb things down. It provided me with the raw signals and symptom data and trusted me to interpret them.

That trust changed everything. Because now, I wasn't guessing. I was investigating.

And for the first time, I was getting **answers**.

4.5   Questioning the paradigm

With journaling back online at full capacity, I set about focusing on debugging my food choices. Patterns emerged almost immediately.

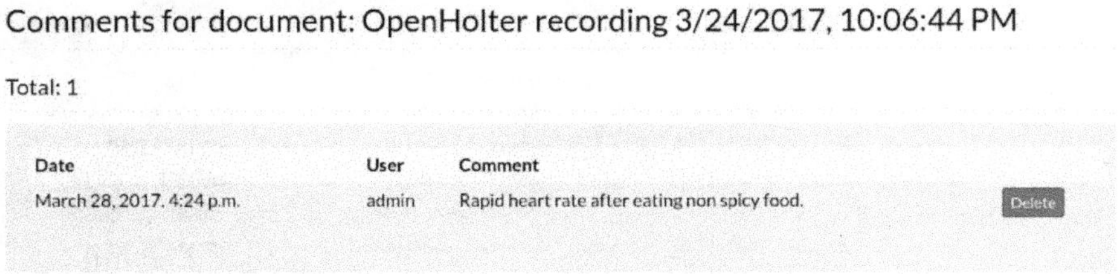

Comments for document: OpenHolter recording 3/24/2017, 10:06:44 PM

Total: 1

Date	User	Comment	
March 28, 2017. 4:24 p.m.	admin	Rapid heart rate after eating non spicy food.	Delete

Fig. 12: Mayan EDMS app view showing the comments of a specific recording.

Meals I thought were "healthy" sent my heart rate variability crashing within minutes. High carbohydrate breakfasts caused arrhythmia. Workouts followed by energy bars triggered an inflammation response. Bread caused delayed dermatitis flare-ups.

On the other hand, consuming fatty cuts of meat and fasting for extended periods without carbohydrates resulted in calm, rhythmic heart signals.

I wasn't guessing. I was **observing**, and I had logs to back it up.

For example, I once tagged a midday snack of fruit and granola as "clean energy". The EKG, however, told a different story; an erratic pattern began just 15 minutes later. Heart stress rose. Atrial flutter. I felt fine, but the data disagreed with me. I repeated this snack three days later. The same heart rhythm disturbance returned along with irritable bowel symptoms.

The data didn't lie. It wasn't emotional. It didn't care about my food philosophy or what fitness influencers had to say. It just told the truth.

So I listened.

Over time, I compiled thousands of correlated entries, including meals, reactions, research papers, symptoms, EKG changes, and other physiological indicators. It became clear that what **others recommended** was often **detrimental to me**. I had my causations.

My "optimal" was **unique, invisible without data**, and **contrary** to conventional nutrition advice I had followed as a martial artist and a health-driven person. Almost every instance I've heard and internalized of *"Everybody knows X is bad"* and *"Everybody knows you have to eat Y to be healthy"* **was incorrect**.

And that was **the breakthrough**.

My gut, heart, inflammation, and energy were all inputs and outputs in one highly individualized system. And I had built the stack to observe, analyze, and adapt it.

In a world obsessed with one-size-fits-all wellness, I was **finding** and **coding my path**. And that path was about to lead me away from decades of dysfunction toward a diet and lifestyle tailored to me.

Not based on dogma. Not based on belief. **Based on data**.

5

DEBUGGING MYSELF

From System Crash to System Reboot

"It is the power of the mind to be unconquerable." - Seneca

In 2016, if someone had asked me to describe what eating healthy looked like, I would have said eating lean meats sparingly, plenty of fruits and vegetables, whole grains, and minimal fat unless it came from a vegetable source. As a martial artist, I believed this was the perfect fuel for high-performance bodies. High energy, low fat, disciplined.

My "healthy" way of eating made my body respond with alarms: **chest palpitations**, **inflammation**, **bloating**, or worse. I'd wake up feeling **groggy**, my **joints ached**. My digestion was **unpredictable**. I was convinced this was just how a high-performance body felt after intense training.

But it turned out that this version of "healthy" was **slowly killing me**.

The OpenHolter alone already provided excellent benefits. Adding Mayan EDMS to the mix multiplied the results. The initial stage of modeling my health was complete. However, I now needed data about other systems.

That's when I reached a common critical juncture: **build** or **buy**.

5.1 Adding more data domains

To continue drilling down my condition and health stack, I needed to add more types of measurements. However, the next round of measurements required more research and development time than that applied to the OpenHolter. To optimize my time and energy, I decided to use what was available and only build or customize when needed. This decision meant that I would have to try out, review, and test a great many other software and devices.

I purchased and tried various products, including smart scales, automatic blood pressure cuffs, blood glucose meters, and smartwatches. And unceremoniously, **I threw many of them away**

I became wary of devices that **awarded badges** or **achievements** instead of focusing on long-term goal setting and sustained improvement. Badges, achievements, and leaderboards are the hallmarks of "gamification", a trend in modern education designed to mimic the engagement strategies of video games. They're everywhere now: in language apps, fitness trackers, and medical courses.

And for good reason: gamification works **at first**.

Rewards, such as badges and point systems, can increase short-term motivation. They create the illusion of momentum. However, the data also reveals something else: like all dopamine hits, the effects are **temporary**.

This phenomenon is known as the "novelty effect". [64] When a new stimulus (like badges) gets introduced, it boosts engagement. But once that novelty fades, so does the motivation. In other words, **the badge becomes the goal, not the learning**.

Another overlooked issue is that gamification systems can unintentionally **infantilize the goal-setting process**. By reducing complex, meaningful learning to a sequence of dopamine hits, they encourage dependency on external validation instead of cultivating resilience, insight, or mastery. This is because gamification influences **behavior** and **attitudes** rather than **results**. [65]

Gamification, when **thoughtfully** designed, can help learners **build momentum** and get enough motivation to **overcome learning curves**. However, it's not a **substitute** for genuine understanding and long-term goals. [66]

As a video game designer and developer, I was acutely aware of these facts, so it was something I strived to avoid when selecting health monitors. [67]

Other products were deeply tied to their software. Using the product meant that vendors would **lock my data** in their system. Unless the data points I obtained were transcendental, it made no sense to keep these devices either.

This selection process enabled me to expand the picture. However, I still validated the results with the OpenHolter and my journal on Mayan EDMS, as they were the only ones I could fully trust. Commercial interests never compromised these results; they were **never sold** or **scrapped to train AI**. My tools never filtered the findings, regardless of how unfavorable they were.

With the selection of the additional devices, I gained a wealth of new information about my body's systems and processes; now, I need to capture detailed information about **my environment** and other factors that were influencing my health but were, for all practical purposes, invisible.

5.2   Monitoring the inside and the outside

Intrigued by the benefits of logging diet and eating patterns, I expanded my scope.

I was now also tracking **sleep patterns**, **VO$_2$ max**, peripheral **oxygen saturation** (SpO$_2$), **body composition**, **bone density**, **visceral fat** level,

blood pressure (BP), **blood sugar**, **urine ketone bodies**, **temporal artery body temperature**, and **body mass index** (BMI).

Of these, **visceral fat** proved to be a reliable biomarker for overall health. Visceral fat is the adipose tissue that accumulates deep inside the **abdominal cavity**, surrounding vital organs like the liver, intestines, and stomach. It differs from subcutaneous fat, which is the fat that can be seen and felt just beneath the skin. This fat accumulation is linked to various health problems, including **heart disease, diabetes**, and **certain cancers**. It also releases inflammatory molecules and fatty acids into the bloodstream, which can negatively impact organ function and increase the risk of disease. [68] [69]

Simply put, visceral fat is a strong, independent predictor of **all-cause mortality** in men. [70]

Since visceral fat directly and indirectly affects waist circumference, this measurement is considered a more accurate predictor of metabolic syndrome than BMI. [71]

Besides adding more body measurements, I also started tracking everything around me. I tested the water I drank for **total dissolved solids** (TDS) and **electrical conductivity** (EC). I even began measuring and logging ambient parameters, including **carbon dioxide** (CO_2) concentration, relative **humidity, temperature**, and **volatile organic compounds** (VOCs).

Improvements to these parameters, such as CO_2 concentration, helped me understand the connection and the immediate effects, like drowsiness. Monitoring and lowering CO_2 concentration allowed me to stay alert more easily and rely less on stimulants, such as coffee or nootropic drinks. [72] [73] [74] It also helped me achieve a more restorative sleep. [75]

Now, entry by entry, I watched as new patterns emerged:

- **Rice?** HRV drops, followed by acid reflux. Increased visceral fat.

- **16-hour fasting window?** More energy all day long. Reduced visceral

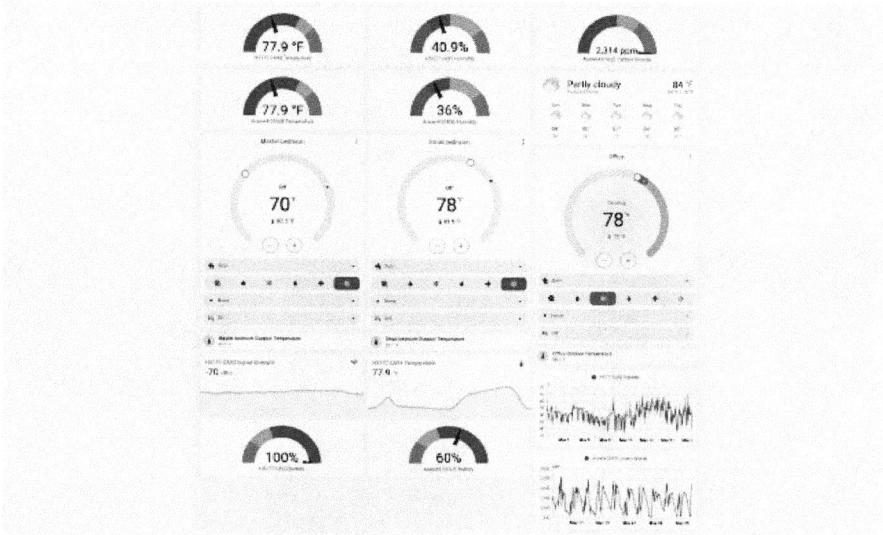

Fig. 1: Climate control and air quality dashboard using Home Assistant.

fat.

- **Oatmeal with fruit?** Immediate gut pain and minor tachycardia.

- **Short workout as I open my eyes?** Lower blood pressure all day. Improved OH.

- **Lean chicken breast?** Felt full but weak, low nutrient density.

- **Lower CO_2?** Alertness. No mental fog.

- **Fatty red meat with eggs?** Calm rhythms. Satiety. No symptoms. Stable blood pressure.

This wasn't guesswork. These were **reproducible** results backed by **timestamped ECG traces** and **symptom tracking**.

*I studied the human metabolism like I would an unfamiliar codebase, rebuilding from **first principles**.*

With my system, I validated that the same meals consistently produced the same reactions. That went against everything I had believed. Against every athlete's meal plan I'd followed. Against the "balanced plate" diagrams I'd internalized since childhood. Athletic dogmas like carbohydrate loading had been destroying me. [76]

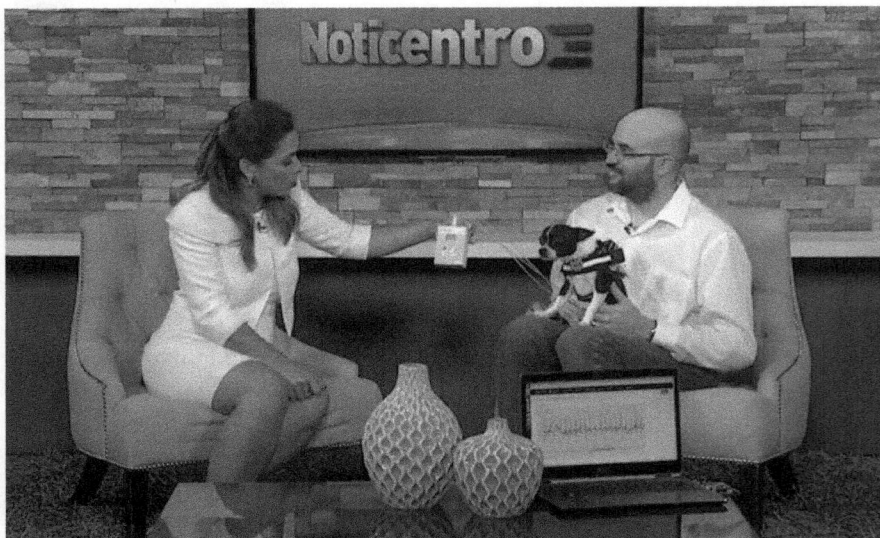

Fig. 2: Interview at WAPA TV, a local network.

5.3   Redefining healthy food

With piles of debugged data, I set out to redefine what healthy food looked like. Mentally, it was hard to accept, but as a developer, I trusted feedback loops. And the feedback was clear: **animal fat** and **animal protein** were healing me; **carbohydrates** and **grains** were hurting me.

So I did what every reasonable engineer does when something's not working: I **refactored**. I redesigned my diet from scratch. Not based on food pyramids or popular health trends but on what the data said my body responded well to.

Gone were the foods that had quietly undermined my well-being.

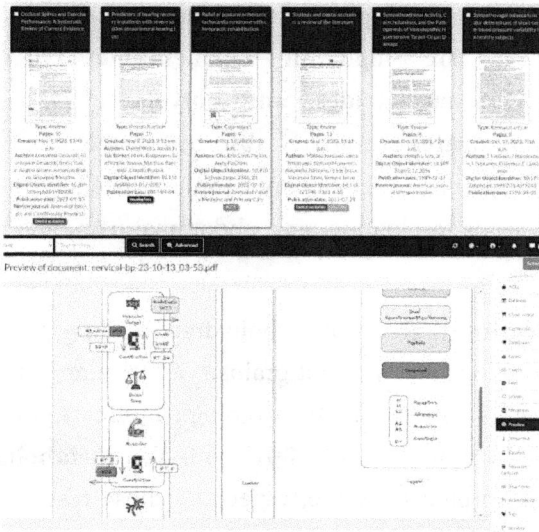

Fig. 3: Local repository of research papers and diagram used to map out the interactions of my conditions.

5.3.1 Grains

Grains were the first to go. Despite their reputation as the foundation of most "balanced diets", whole grains consistently left me **bloated**, **sluggish**, and **inflamed**. For decades, I consumed them without question, accepting them as a cornerstone of good nutrition. However, when I started monitoring my symptoms and comparing them with my diet, a clear pattern emerged. Whether it was brown rice, quinoa, or whole wheat bread, the result was invariably the same.

This general sense of malaise, I later discovered, is **not uncommon**. Grains and grain-derived products, even those marketed as health foods, such as soy milk, contain **phytic acid**, a compound that binds essential minerals like iron, calcium, manganese, and zinc. This binding process, known as **chelation**, forms **insoluble** complexes that the gut cannot absorb, leading to their excretion. As a result, the bioavailability of these critical nutrients is

drastically reduced. [77]

But the issue doesn't end with phytic acid. Many grains, particularly wheat, rye, and barley, are high in **Fermentable Oligosaccharides, Disaccharides, Monosaccharides, and Polyols** (FODMAPs). These short-chain **carbohydrates** are poorly absorbed in the small intestine and tend to ferment in the colon. For many people, especially those with IBS, this fermentation leads to bloating, gas, abdominal pain, and altered bowel habits. [78]

Then come the **lectins**, a group of carbohydrate-binding proteins found in many plants, including legumes and grains. While plants use lectins as a **defense** mechanism against pests, their biological effects in humans are far more complex. Lectins can **interfere** with the **metabolism** of lipids, carbohydrates, and proteins. Some, especially those resistant to heat and digestion, bind to the **gut lining**, impairing nutrient absorption and contributing to **increased intestinal permeability**. They've been shown to affect gut epithelial cells, alter the microbiome composition, modulate immune function, and disrupt normal hormonal signaling. Certain lectins have also been linked to **inflammation, organ enlargement, organ atrophy**, and **metabolic disturbances**. [79] [80]

Because of these effects, lectins are sometimes classified as **antinutrients** and even **toxins**. While some lectins can be deactivated by proper cooking or fermentation, others persist despite standard food preparation methods, particularly those found in grains and legumes that are consumed in large quantities. [81]

5.3.2   Cereals

Cereals, once a ubiquitous presence at my breakfast table and a go-to snack for movie nights, were triggering the same symptoms I had come to associate with grains: bloating, brain fog, headaches, and inflammation. More surprisingly, I began to notice a decline in **cognitive performance**. Over several weeks, I tracked my productivity on days with and without cereal consumption, and the pattern was hard to ignore. My work output declined in quantity, and the mental effort required to produce it increased.

When I began researching the health effects of breakfast cereals, especially **ready-to-eat** varieties, I was struck by how difficult it was to find **reliable**, **independent** data. Much of the available literature is clouded by industry influence or focuses narrowly on metrics such as fiber content. Instead of being grounded in rigorous science, the foundation of cereal as a dietary staple appears more closely tied to **ideological** beliefs and early 20th-century health movements. [82]

What shocked me even more was how the very phrases used to promote these products today **echo** the same language used when the Kellogg Company, founded by Will Keith Kellogg, brother of Dr. John Harvey Kellogg, introduced its cornflakes brand nearly **120** years ago. Consider these vintage advertisements:

- *"And the difference is one that you will like and never tire of - that will be good for you no matter how much you eat."* - (1906, October 19). The Gazette, p. 7. City: Cedar Rapids, Iowa [83]

- *"And you can eat your fill without fear of harmful results."* - (1906, October 18). The Courier, p. 7. City: Waterloo, Iowa [84]

- *"Start the day on the right food and you will think - you will think easier, more clearly - all day long."* - (1907, January 12). The Philadelphia Inquirer, p. 6. City: Philadelphia, Pennsylvania [85]

These lines mirror today's marketing, which continues to present cereals as wholesome, energizing, and essential. Modern strategies go even further, employing **psychological tactics** such as character **archetypes** and **gamified experiences** to build brand **loyalty in children**, instilling in them an **emotional bond** with breakfast cereals. [86] [87]

So powerful is this **conditioning** that we've internalized the idea that certain foods belong at specific times of day. We've been reprogrammed to follow eating habits shaped by "meal timing" bias and perceptions of what's considered "appropriate" for each meal. We don't just eat "breakfast"; we eat "breakfast foods". This mindset has dramatically **reduced** variety and limited the inclusion of **nutrient-dense** foods. [88] [89] [90]

Instead of a nourishing first meal, we've mainly replaced breakfast with processed, sugar-laden products that lack strong evidence of long-term benefit for most people. [91] [92]

Breaking free from the "breakfast food" paradigm has been transformative. I now happily start my mornings with meals like **steak**, **eggs**, and **avocado**, a far cry from the cartoon-branded, sugar-filled boxes of my past.

5.3.3 Sugar

Sugar quickly emerged as a major culprit. Once I began tracking my glucose responses and HRV patterns, the spike-and-crash rhythm became unmistakable. It wasn't just about weight gain or dental issues. Sugar seemed to actively impair my cognitive clarity, destabilize my mood, and trigger latent inflammation. Even small amounts could disrupt my metabolic equilibrium for hours, and my thinking would become erratic. In my system, sugar was like **noise** I was trying to eliminate.

But as with cereals, finding **reliable** research on sugar and sugar-sweetened beverages proved difficult. The integrity of the data itself has become a **subject** of investigation. Systematic reviews examining this statistical bias have revealed a disturbing trend: studies funded by the sugar-sweetened beverage industry were **five times** more likely to report no association between sugary drinks and obesity compared to studies independently funded. [93] [94] [95]

This isn't just a matter of oversight; it points to deeper systemic problems. The food pyramid, long upheld as a trusted dietary guide, was shaped more by **weak science** and **corporate lobbying** than by solid nutritional evidence. [96] [97] [98]

Even artificial sweeteners, once promoted as harmless sugar substitutes, have been associated with **insulin resistance**, impaired **glucose regulation, metabolic syndrome, reduced satiety**, altered **gut microbiota**, and the **obesity epidemic**. Some studies even report heightened **cardiometabolic risk** associated with regular consumption of artificial sweeteners. [99] [100] [101]

One truth became impossible to ignore: while **salt** is **essential** to life, **sugar is not**. Reframing sugar as an unnecessary agent of metabolic disruption allowed me to break free from its **biological** and **psychologically** addictive grip. [102] [103] [104]

5.3.4 Starches

Starches, such as potatoes and cassava, turned out not to be good either. These "safe carbs", long considered acceptable even in strict diets, triggered sharp blood sugar spikes and gut discomfort. Far from slow-burn fuels, they behaved like **metabolic landmines**. The bloating and post-meal fatigue left no doubt: even unprocessed starches didn't agree with my biology.

Starches were a **frustratingly hard** topic to research. Few studies directly investigate the impact of different starch types on body weight, metabolic markers, or individual health. Instead, much of the literature compares starch-rich diets against ultra-processed or sugar-laden alternatives, creating a **misleading** contrast. It felt like **price anchoring**, a **cognitive bias** where a poor baseline (junk food) makes the alternative (starch) appear better than it is. Although anchoring is a common practice in marketing, its psychological mechanism also applies to biased research framing. [105]

But I wasn't looking for the lesser of two evils; I wanted what worked for my body.

A troubling pattern emerged: conflicts of interest were **common**, and the topic was often deemed "controversial", especially when diet and obesity were involved. It became clear that nutrition research is a **minefield**, and many researchers **play it safe** to avoid antagonizing powerful industry sponsors. [106]

When studies do highlight adverse outcomes, they typically focus on refined starches. These are rapidly digested, causing **sharp spikes** in **glucose** and **insulin** levels, followed by precipitous drops that trigger **fatigue, irritability**, and **hunger**. Refined starches are strongly linked to **insulin resistance, metabolic syndrome, cognitive impairment**, and rising **type 2 diabetes** rates. [107] [108] [109]

Of course, not all starches are the same. When research becomes accessible, it usually focuses on a narrow category: **resistant starch** (RS). RS is a type of starch that resists digestion in the small intestine and ferments in the colon. It is often praised for its lower glycemic impact, but studies rarely explore the potential **drawbacks** of RS.

RS isn't inherently good, it is just less harmful than refined starches. Even though RS leads to smaller glucose increases, those increases **still** occurred, and I didn't want or need them.

Worse still, RS fermentation alters the **microbiome**. It encourages bacteria rich in **carbohydrate-active enzymes** (CAZymes), especially those belonging to the **Bacteroidota** family, which possess sophisticated **starch-utilization systems** (Sus). These can dominate, reducing microbial **diversity** and increasing the risk of **dysbiosis**. [110] [111] [112]

Bacteroides species are highly complex and adaptable; they can **manipulate** their environment and even the host immune system to **outcompete** other microbes. Clinically, when they are outside of the gut, they're implicated in serious anaerobic infections and carry high mortality rates (>19%). [113]

Their genomes are loaded with **antibiotic-resistance genes**, and they're prolific in **horizontal gene transfer** (HGT), sharing resistance traits with other gut bacteria. [114] [115] [116] Species like Bacteroides thetaiotaomicron are especially adept at **evading antibiotics**. [117]

If microbial shifts weren't concerning enough, high-starch diets also

exacerbate non-alcoholic fatty liver disease (NAFLD) by promoting de novo lipogenesis and increasing fatty acid flow into the liver. [118]

In contrast, low- or no-starch diets have been shown to **improve gut health** and **boost microbiome diversity**. [119]

The choice became crystal clear: starches were out.

5.3.5   Bread

Bread, regardless of how artisanal, proved to be another culprit.   I experimented with various grains and preparation methods, including gluten-free options, yet chest palpitations, gut disturbances, and dermatitis persisted.   Sourdough was the **sole exception**, but even then, its high carbohydrate content limited my intake to rare, small portions.

Wheat can also cause harm **without** even being eaten.   Bakers and others who frequently handle flour may develop **irritant contact dermatitis**, also known as **irritant contact eczema**, due to occupational exposure to flour. [120]

While celiac disease is often viewed as the primary cause of gluten-related issues, the reality is more complex. A significant rise in gluten consumption has paralleled an **increase** in celiac disease among children, suggesting that **exposure** may be driving this epidemic. [121] Undiagnosed celiac disease carries a nearly **fourfold** (4x) increase in mortality risk and has become dramatically more prevalent over the past **50** years. [122]

You don't have to have celiac disease to experience negative effects from bread. Two decades ago, celiac was considered rare, but today, more people follow gluten-free diets than can be explained by diagnosed or extrapolated number of cases.   This trend has led to a formal **reclassification** of gluten-related disorders, including **wheat allergy**, **dermatitis herpetiformis**, **gluten ataxia**, and **non-celiac gluten sensitivity**. [123] [124]

A common assertion is that modern wheat is uniquely inflammatory. While selective breeding has increased certain **gluten epitopes** known to trigger celiac disease, gluten has **always** been a natural component of wheat. [125] Some evidence suggests that heirloom varieties may contain fewer epitopes; however, the clinical safety and health benefits of these varieties remain unproven.

The reality is that **modification** has **overtaken** wheat agriculture. The development of high-yield semi-dwarf wheat in the mid-20th century reshaped global agriculture.

In the mid-**1940s**, Mexican farming was notoriously **unproductive**, and the country was on the **brink of famine**.

In **1944**, Norman E. Borlaug, an agricultural scientist, began work with the **Rockefeller Foundation's Mexican Agricultural Program** (MAP) to improve wheat yields. His disease-resistant, semi-dwarf wheat varieties helped Mexico become self-sufficient in wheat by **1956**. For this and other contributions in the field of plant-based food supply, Borlaug won the 1970 Nobel Peace Prize. [126] [127]

These new wheat strains were also **higher** in gluten content, as gluten is important for seedling robustness and yield. The wheat that Borlaug developed is a "semi-dwarf" variety, which resists "lodging", meaning it doesn't fall over easily in wind or hail. This characteristic made it **highly attractive** and contributed significantly to its rapid growth and **widespread** adoption. [128]

As these varieties spread, gluten sensitivity **rose dramatically** in regions where Borlaug's wheat was adopted. Countries like Mexico experienced sharp increases in **obesity** and **gluten-related disorders**, conditions that were previously **rare**. [129] [130] [131] By the **1960s**, scientists also observed a **decline** in wheat's **mineral density**, which coincided with the introduction of these high-yield cultivars. [132]

In summary, selective breeding for agricultural yield has dramatically transformed wheat, boosting gluten and epitopes that contribute to gluten-related disorders **globally** while also reducing its mineral content.

As much as I love bread, the health risks far outweigh any benefits beyond taste and texture. I can now count on **two hands** how many times a **year** I eat it.

My findings about the health effects of sugar, grains, and other plant-based foods aren't isolated; they echo a broader, often **buried** reality in nutrition science, complicated by **bias** and **controversy**. [133]

On Earth, at least, living organisms have a persistent tendency **not** to want **to die**, and plants are **no exception**. Unlike animals, which can flee or fight back, plants are rooted and rely on chemicals for defense. Plants don't just use chemicals for defense; they wage full-on **chemical warfare**. We must realize that their survival strategies take into account a life cycle and time span that are vastly different from our own; they are in it for the long haul and the well-being of their entire species. They aim to eliminate both the **immediate** and **long-term** threats to their survival.

From **toxins** to **mycorrhizal signaling networks**, plant life is **far** more biologically and chemically complex than we ever consider when we eat them. [134] [135]

With that awareness, I stopped viewing plants as inherently **benign**. I recognized them as living entities, genetically equipped to survive by **any means**.

With harmful foods eliminated, I began to embrace the meals that consistently restored my energy, clarity, and balance, meal after meal.

5.3.6 Eggs

Eggs, once vilified for their cholesterol content, became a staple in my diet. Every morning I started with eggs, I noticed consistent metabolic stability. They provided satiety and strength with minimal digestive effort, keeping my energy level steady for hours. These aren't just breakfast items; they are performance-enhancing biomolecules wrapped in a shell.

Furthermore, eggs are a nutritional powerhouse: rich in **high-quality protein, essential amino acids, vitamins,** and **minerals,** including **choline** and **lutein.** Choline supports **brain** development and **liver** function, while lutein plays a crucial role in maintaining **cognitive health** and **protecting the eyes.** Research now suggests that lutein may help guard against **age-related cognitive decline** across the **lifespan.** [136] [137]

Eggs aren't just nutrient-dense; they may actively protect health across the lifespan. Beyond being a superior protein source, eggs contain bioactive compounds that have been shown to support **antioxidant defense, antimicrobial** and **antihypertensive** effects, **immune modulation,** and **metabolic regulation.** Egg proteins and lipids have been proven to have protective effects on **cardiovascular health, brain function,** and even **cancer prevention.** [138] [139]

Eggs were once demonized because of **cholesterol,** but science has moved on. Multiple studies now demonstrate that dietary cholesterol from eggs does **not** adversely affect blood cholesterol levels in most individuals. On the contrary, eggs **improve** lipid profiles, **increasing HDL** ("good" cholesterol) without significantly affecting LDL when included in a healthy diet. When **combined** with a **low-carbohydrate** approach, eggs help maintain or enhance metabolic markers, **raising HDL-C** levels, **lowering triglycerides,** reducing **blood pressure,** improving **fasting glucose** levels, and decreasing **visceral fat,** all without increasing LDL-C. [140]

Egg cholesterol isn't merely harmless; it's biologically **essential.** Cholesterol is a **precursor** to steroid hormones, vitamin D synthesis, and cell membrane integrity. [141]

Looking back, I regret how long I avoided eggs, how often I tossed the **yolks,** and how readily I reached for ultra-processed powdered egg replacements that **masqueraded** as healthier options.

5.3.7 Organ meat

Organ meat was next. Initially, I approached it cautiously, like medicine, in small amounts. But what I discovered surprised me. It was like flipping a switch on nutrient density. My stamina and metabolic markers noticeably improved once I incorporated them into my diet. My body seemed to respond exceptionally well to liver, almost as if it had been waiting for it.

Organ meats, particularly liver, are among the **most** nutrient-dense foods available. Because the liver performs hundreds of vital metabolic functions in animals, it **accumulates** exceptionally high concentrations of **essential micronutrients**. It is especially rich in B-complex vitamins, particularly **B12** and **folate**, as well as **iron, zinc, copper**, and **selenium**. Liver also supplies generous amounts of **fat-soluble vitamins** A, D, E, and K. It is a complete source of high-quality protein, making it, in many ways, **nature's original multivitamin**. [142] [143]

Emerging research also suggests that organ meat consumption may be **inversely associated** with non-alcoholic fatty liver disease (NAFLD). A 2023 study revealed that a higher intake of organ meats like liver and kidney was linked to a significantly **lower** prevalence of non-alcoholic steatohepatitis (NASH), the more severe inflammatory subtype of NAFLD. [144]

Another underappreciated nutrient in organ meats is **selenium**, a trace mineral essential for **thyroid hormone synthesis, antioxidant defense**, and maintaining a **healthy immune** system. Some traditional sausage preparations that include organ meats can be excellent dietary sources of selenium. [145]

The consequences of selenium **deficiency** can be profound. It has been linked to **cardiovascular disease**, increased susceptibility to **infections**, and, in extreme cases, to two life-threatening endemic diseases: **Keshan disease** and **Kashin-Beck disease** (KBD). Keshan disease, in particular, has a mortality rate exceeding **80%** if left untreated. [146] [147]

I had never liked organ meats before; even the smell could trigger nausea. However, I came to understand that this aversion was primarily **psychological**, shaped by years of **marketing, cultural** avoidance, and lack of **familiarity**. Most of us grew up associating organ meats with poverty or the past, not performance or health.

Thankfully, there are ways to enjoy the nutritional benefits of organ meats while your palate adapts. Freeze-dried liver capsules are one convenient option. A more integrative culinary approach involves blending small amounts of finely minced liver into ground beef, meatballs, burger patties, or sausages, a traditional cooking technique used to enhance both nutrition and flavor subtly.

Once I studied the health benefits and understood their value, my relationship with organ meats underwent a significant change. They became not only acceptable but **foundational**.

5.3.8 Bone broth

Bone broth, something I once dismissed as an old wives' remedy, became a trusted foundation for my well-being. Whether recovering from illness, emerging from a fast, or simply seeking warmth on a chilly day, a bowl of bone broth soothed my gut, provided steady hydration and electrolytes, and offered gentle, grounding nourishment.

Bone broth is made by simmering animal bones and connective tissues for hours, a process that extracts **collagen, gelatin, amino acids** (like glycine), and **trace minerals**.

Traditionally used during convalescence, the practice of consuming bone broth and its other benefits are now supported by emerging **scientific evidence**.

A recent open-label clinical trial of the Bone Broth Diet, conducted in obese adults undergoing **two 3-week** intermittent fasting cycles, revealed an average weight loss of **4.8 kg** in the first cycle and **2.6 kg** in the second.

Participants also showed improvements in **blood glucose** levels, **waist circumference**, **cardiometabolic** and **psychological** health, as well as **appetite regulation**, while maintaining quality of life. [148]

But bone broth's benefits extend well beyond weight loss.

Autoimmune diseases, such as **multiple sclerosis, lupus, Crohn's disease**, and **Hashimoto's thyroiditis**, were once considered **strictly genetic**. That belief stems mainly from the Nobel Prize-winning clonal selection theory of the **1960s**, which showed that rogue lymphocytes could cause autoimmunity. [149]

However, the concordance rate for autoimmune conditions among identical twins rarely exceeds **75%**, suggesting that **environmental** or **epigenetic** factors also play a significant role. [150] This perspective still includes the human genome but also overlooks the complex **microbiome** of the gut, particularly bacteria within the Bacteroidota phylum, which exhibit remarkable **genomic** and **epigenetic complexity**. These microbes have a profound influence on **immune function, metabolism**, and the integrity of the **gut barrier**. [151] [152] [153] [154]

More recent research has identified **intestinal permeability**, often referred to as "leaky gut", as a key mechanism linking **gut health** and **autoimmunity**. **Zonulin**, the **only** known physiological regulator of tight junctions in the gut, plays a central role. When overexpressed in genetically susceptible individuals, it can lead to a **compromised** gut barrier and trigger **immune dysregulation**. [155]

Once dismissed as **myth** and **pseudoscience**, "leaky gut syndrome" is now taken seriously in **immunology** and **gastroenterology**. Animal models and clinical studies show that modulating zonulin and restoring barrier integrity can help **prevent** or **treat** autoimmune conditions. [156] [157] [158] [159] [160] [161]

Disrupted gut barriers are also implicated in **IBD, IBS, metabolic disorders**, and **inflammatory joint** or **neurodegenerative diseases**. The common thread is gut barrier dysfunction, often coupled with **dysbiosis** and individual genetic or epigenetic vulnerabilities. [162]

Even COVID-19 research **supports** this connection. Studies show that gut microbiota **composition** correlates with disease **severity**. Many patients experienced GI symptoms, and post-COVID dysbiosis may contribute to long-COVID symptoms, underscoring the microbiome's systemic influence. [163] [164]

Key nutrients in bone broth may help **restore** gut lining integrity and support nutrient absorption. Contemporary reviews confirm the value of bone broth as a functional food for gut health, particularly in conditions related to **inflammation** and **permeability**. [165]

In this light, bone broth becomes more than a recovery tool: it's a nutrient-dense, mineral-rich **elixir** that supports **hydration**, **gut repair**, and **immune resilience**. Its electrolytes make it especially helpful during fasting, illness, or daily upkeep.

5.3.9 Red meat

Red meat was the game changer. It delivered results that **no plant-based food had ever achieved**. My iron levels normalized. My HRV increased. Post-meal fatigue vanished. I could go for **hours** without feeling hungry or experiencing cravings. Contrary to decades of dietary dogma, red meat didn't burden my system; it **repaired** it. The more I tracked my progress, the more obvious it became: red meat wasn't the problem; it was a big part of the **solution**.

When I prioritized red meat, the improvements went far beyond lab results. They showed up in how I felt, moved, and slept. Scrapes healed **faster**, muscle recovery after workouts **accelerated**, and my sleep became **deeper** and more **restorative**. For the first time in years, my energy felt stable and effortless.

As with other foods I investigated, the literature and research around red meat are often **skewed**, frequently based on **agendas** other than nutritional inquiry.

166 167 168

Red meat ranks among the most **effective** foods for preserving and rebuilding muscle, especially during recovery or aging. Numerous studies have confirmed that a higher protein intake from red meat supports **muscle protein synthesis** and enhances strength and function in adults, particularly when combined with resistance training. [169]

For decades, red meat became the **scapegoat** behind chronic disease. That fear dates back to Ancel Keys's **1950s** "lipid-heart" hypothesis, which **selectively** used data to link saturated fat to heart disease while **dismissing** conflicting evidence. The result? A half-century of **misplaced** blame on red meat and saturated animal fat. [170]

However, recent meta-analyses and reviews have **dismantled** that narrative. There is **no strong evidence** that saturated fat from unprocessed sources, such as red meat, increases the risk of heart disease. Indeed, large-scale reviews suggest that adults **maintain** their current levels of red meat intake, citing **low-quality evidence** for any **significant harm**. [171] [172]

Even more compelling is the **absence** of disease in traditional red-meat-eating cultures, such as the **Maasai**, the **Inuit**, or certain **Argentine** communities, where heart disease was historically **rare** despite high consumption of saturated fats. Research on the topic is scarce, but when it does emerge, scientists often attribute these health outcomes to other lifestyle factors and claim that these additional factors are not found in Western society. When these factors are observed in Western society, such as **calorie restriction**, **intermittent fasting**, **physical activity**, and **energy expenditure**, the definition of the factor is taken to the extreme in a practice of reductio ad absurdum to disqualify it as reproducible. [173]

A high-protein diet is an **effective** and **safe** tool for weight loss that can help prevent obesity and its associated diseases. High-protein diet energy expenditure increase involves two aspects: first, proteins have a markedly higher **diet-induced thermogenesis** (DIT) than carbohydrates and fats.

Second, protein intake helps prevent a decrease in **fat-free mass** (FFM), which in turn helps maintain resting energy expenditure despite weight loss. [174]

Eight weeks of a high-protein, omega-3-enriched diet combined with exercise **decreased** circulating anti-inflammatory markers and pro-inflammatory markers (PBMC) in men. A high-protein diet **attenuated** anti-inflammatory markers on gene expression levels in PBMC. [175]

This journey, which went from questioning the merits and persecution of red meat to fully embracing it, taught me something profound: red meat is not a cardiovascular **threat** but a **cornerstone of recovery**. Now, I feast on red meat almost daily. Whether a fatty **ribeye**, a budget-friendly **chuck steak**, or a hearty serving of **ground beef**, a portion of red meat is always part of my plate. Red meat isn't just a choice; it's become a form of **metabolic therapy**.

5.3.10   Fish

Fish, particularly oily varieties like sardines and salmon, brought calmness to my system. These meals produced smoother HRV curves and an uplifted mood. Even small portions of these types of fish left me feeling full and satisfied but without any bloating.

Marine omega-3 fats, such as **Eicosapentaenoic acid** (EPA) and **Docosahexaenoic acid** (DHA), are known to **reduce** resting heart rate and **increase** HRV, a key biomarker of autonomic flexibility. In clinical studies, even **modest doses** of DHA-rich fish oil have been proven to reduce heart rate and improve HRV significantly. This improvement was observed not just in healthy adults but also in overweight individuals. These remarkable shifts were evident in my own HRV data: after consuming sardine meals, my HRV traces became noticeably less erratic and more resilient. [176 177 178 179]

High fish consumption is associated with **lower** rates of **depression**. Mechanisms include strengthening **neuronal membrane function**, reducing **neuroinflammation**, and modulating **serotonin** and other **neurotransmitter** systems. [180]

Regular consumption of oily fish shows a link to a **lower** risk of **cardiovascular mortality** and a **reduced** likelihood of **ischemic events**. Benefits include improved **myocardial efficiency**, enhanced **endothelial function**, and a better balance of **sympathetic** and **parasympathetic** balance. [181] [182]

I swapped quick, processed snack bars for a can of sardines. When I'm short on time, a single serving of sardines supplies the right nutrition to power me through until my next meal.

5.3.11   Dairy

Dairy, especially full-fat and fermented varieties, was another surprising win.   Growing up, I was told dairy was either essential or dangerous, depending entirely on the decade.   For years, I wrestled with both **hypocalcemia** and **hypercalciuria**, conditions I eventually connected to a persistent, **low-grade metabolic acidosis**. One clinician even blamed it squarely on mass-market pasteurized milk. So, I was hesitant to add dairy to my diet. Carefully reintroducing thoughtfully sourced full-fat dairy, such as **ghee, grass-fed butter, kefir, Greek yogurt**, and **aged cheese**, transformed everything.

Fermented dairy is rich in **enzymes, bioactive peptides**, and **fat-soluble vitamins** like K2, yet low in lactose.   It also contains **butyric acid, conjugated linoleic acid** (CLA), and **lactoferrin**, which support mineral balance, gut integrity, immune function, and steadier post-meal glucose levels.   I carefully tracked the improvements from fermented dairy in my symptom logs and wellness data, and the results were undeniable.

Clinical evidence backed what I observed.

A randomized controlled trial found that overweight women who added 30 g/day of milk protein concentrate (MPC) to a calorie-restricted diet over 8 weeks experienced **significant** improvements in **BMI, waist circumference, fat mass, fasting glucose** levels, **insulin levels, LDL** levels, and **leptin** levels while increasing **HDL** and **adiponectin** levels. [183]

A **2010** randomized trial demonstrated that adding milk during weight loss blunted typical spikes in hunger and **food cravings**. [184]

A **2020** systematic review showed that consuming >**1.2 g** protein/kg/day consistently enhanced feelings of fullness and satiety in overweight or obese individuals. [185] [186]

More recently, a **2023** crossover study found that a dairy-based, high-protein breakfast (~30 g) significantly boosted **satiety** and reduced **hunger** in overweight women before lunch. [187]

These effects align with my experience tracking HRV, meal-time glucose, and bowel symptom trends.

Like fats and cholesterol, I've been told all my life that dairy products like cheese and butter were bad for me. Now, I can't imagine myself eating a steak without a thick slab of butter melting on top of it, especially the one my wife makes at home.

Dairy products are nowadays an **essential** part of my **daily protein quota**.

5.3.12   Fermented vegetables

Fermented vegetables, once merely an afterthought, transformed into a strategic linchpin in my diet. **Sauerkraut, kimchi**, and traditionally **fermented cucumbers** offered a potent probiotic boost, stabilizing digestion and seamlessly counteracting the heaviness of fatty meals. Remarkably, even **modest, intermittent** servings yielded subtle yet profound benefits: diminished bloating, more consistent bowel movements, and a refreshed lightness after eating. These fermented foods became especially vital in the periods **before** and **after** my emergency surgery, playing a central role in bolstering my **gut resilience** and **accelerating** my recovery. [188] [189]

These foods deliver **live cultures**, primarily **lactic acid bacteria** (LAB), along with bioactive **metabolites** that help stabilize digestion, particularly when paired with **fatty meals**. Unlike probiotic pills, only small, intermittent servings were needed. The impact of fermented vegetables on bloating, regularity, and digestive "lightness" was subtle but tangible. [190] [191]

Beyond the gut, fermented vegetables even enhance **mental** wellness through the **gut-brain axis**, mediating **stress response**, **cognition**, and **mood**, courtesy of **bidirectional** communication between gut microbes and brain chemistry. [192]

Fermentation also pre-digests complex **carbohydrates** and **cellulose**, freeing **micronutrients** and boosting the **bioavailability of vitamins** B, K_2, and C. This process generates **postbiotics**, including **lactic acid** and **short-chain fatty acids** (SCFAs), that support **gut barrier integrity**, which is **crucial** following surgery. Sauerkraut extract was shown to protect intestinal cells more effectively than raw cabbage, likely due to the presence of these compounds. [193]

Fermented veggies gave me the benefits of fresh produce without the downsides. They're **affordable, shelf-stable**, and **safe**. For me, they have been a nutritional complement to my diet and crucial amid surgical recovery.

In addition to these dietary changes, I also reexamined the way I was **consuming** them. I also realized my reliance on processed food as a way to shorten meal preparation time was a **grave** mistake, as I've been exchanging time and convenience for **increased mortality**. [194]

I now strive to eat food with minimal preparation or none, if possible. The final product I eat should resemble the raw material from which it is made.

Continuing to learn not just about the food's composition but also how the body absorbs it, I moved on to metabolism next. I studied the human metabolism like I would an unfamiliar codebase, rebuilding from **first principles**. I was breaking down a problem into its most basic, fundamental elements and then rebuilding it from scratch based on those truths rather than relying on assumptions or conventional wisdom.

This approach provided me with a **fresh perspective**, enabled **innovative solutions**, and led to **breakthroughs**.

5.4   Eating patterns

In addition to the new food items, I began experimenting with eating patterns to test the ingrained sports dogma that dictated I needed to eat every two hours. I started allowing my body to speak, to **tell me** when and how much to consume.

It wasn't a sudden shift but a gradual recalibration. Some days, three meals felt right; others, a single, hefty brunch paired with a midday snack. Some days, I would go on an empty stomach and just have a satisfying dinner. I stopped **forcing** myself to fill the void, to meet some **arbitrary** expectation of fullness. Remarkably, I became **attuned** to my body's **hunger signals** in ways I never thought possible.

Then came one particular day. I was utterly immersed in a project, drinking only electrolytes and a few cups of bone broth. The next day, the same pattern repeated. By the third day, a startling realization hit me: I hadn't consumed any **solid food** for **forty-eight** hours. And yet, I didn't feel hungry or weak, quite the opposite. I possessed an unusual surge of **energy** and **focus**, and the work I accomplished in those forty-eight hours would have usually taken twice as long. It took me a while to truly accept that the human body possessed the remarkable capacity to **sustain** itself for **more** than a day without food. I'd previously considered extended fasting a reckless activity. So, with an open mind, I began researching, delving into the science behind it.

My investigation led me to the concept of **autophagy**. The term "autophagy" is derived from the Latin words for "self" and "eating". While that might sound scary, autophagy is a self-renewal mechanism that **degrades** and **recycles** cellular components to maintain the stability of the intracellular environment and the cell's ability to cope with unfavorable conditions.

Specifically, during physiological stress, autophagy acts as an **anti-infection** shield, actively suppressing the inflammatory response and preventing irreparable tissue damage. Furthermore, autophagy in vascular endothelial cells **promotes** wound **angiogenesis**, a process that involves the formation of new blood vessels to deliver vital oxygen and nutrients to the healing area. [195]

It appears that **not eating** may lead to **improved healing**. Many of my childhood memories now made sense. When sick, I would just lie in bed, not wanting to eat anything. The only meal I wholeheartedly desired was my mother's chicken soup. After three days of consuming just that soup, I was right as rain. My body was telling me that it wanted to remain in an autophagic state.

However, autophagy isn't simply a tool for recovering from the flu or for weight loss; it's an **essential** process for good health. Defects in autophagy are linked to a startling array of diseases: **neurodegenerative conditions** like Alzheimer's and Parkinson's, **cardiomyopathy**, **tumorigenesis**, **diabetes**, **fatty liver disease**, and even **Crohn's disease**. [196]

Extended fasting isn't a fleeting trend or a restrictive diet; it's an activity that demonstrably leads to **better health** and, potentially, **increased longevity**.

Autophagy research **isn't new**. The initial groundwork was laid back in **1955** when the first component of the process was discovered. Over the decades, a growing body of research has steadily expanded our understanding of the biological intricacies of this process. Then, in **1993**, Yoshinori Ohsumi, a professor at the Tokyo Institute of Technology, made groundbreaking discoveries, identifying many of the steps and molecular tools involved in this complex recycling mechanism. For these contributions, he received the **2016 Nobel Prize in Physiology or Medicine**. [197] [198]

With that validation, I started doing **intermittent fasting**, [199] **time-restricted eating**, [200] and **One Meal A Day** (OMAD). [201]

Within weeks, I felt the difference:

- **Brain fog?** Gone.

- **Acid reflux?** Vanished.

- **Skin rashes?** Cleared.

- **Migraines?** Disappeared.

- **IBS?** A thing of the past.

- **Chronic fatigue?** No more.

- **Fatty liver markers?** Normalized.

- **Joint pain?** Nonexistent.

- **Morning energy?** Surging.

- **Right Lower Quadrant (RLQ) pain?** Improved significantly.

As my various conditions slowly began to fade, one symptom persisted: my nagging (RLQ) pain. It wasn't as excruciating as it once was; I'd decreased its perceived pain rating from a **7 out of 10** to a mere whisper at **1**. This lone lingering symptom was a bit ominous. Its occasional return made me wonder what was still **lurking beneath** the surface. However, after achieving a **90% improvement** in this long-term condition, I was thrilled.

5.5 New insights

I didn't just feel better; **I had proof**. With each round of changes, my EKG showed increasingly stronger and steadier patterns. The resting heart rate **dropped**, and HRV **increased**.

HRV is a very significant indicator of health. It describes the natural variation in the time interval **between** heartbeats. The time between each heartbeat is **not perfectly consistent**, and these slight variations are normal and healthy.

A high HRV indicates that the body can maintain a balance between the **parasympathetic** and **sympathetic** nervous systems. It is linked to better **stress management**, **faster recovery** from physical activity, and a **reduced risk** of chronic diseases. [202]

These heart rate fluctuations are undetectable except with specialized devices. If it weren't for the long-term observation system I've developed using the OpenHolter and Mayan EDMS, I would never have been able to utilize this vital parameter to fine-tune my health. I would not have even been **aware** of its existence!

5.6 More benefits

My improvements were not exclusive to my cardiovascular system; I also experienced overwhelming improvements in other conditions.

Inflammatory markers faded. My sleep improved in depth and efficiency. My gut started to heal quietly and steadily. Post-meal cramping and unpredictable bathroom emergencies became history, replaced by calm digestion and regularity. Once a system was debugged and started working better, it helped other systems return to nominal function.

The foods I once avoided, such as **saturated fats**, **cholesterol**, and **red meat**, turned out to be exactly what my body needed to recover. What I thought was hurting me was helping me heal. This wasn't just a nutritional change. This was **system recovery**.

The engineer in me kept testing, iterating, and logging. The former martial artist in me adjusted training routines to support my new energy rhythms. And the patient in me? He finally **stopped suffering**.

When you discover and understand what your body truly needs and craves, and you trust the data, it's no longer a diet; **it's newfound freedom**.

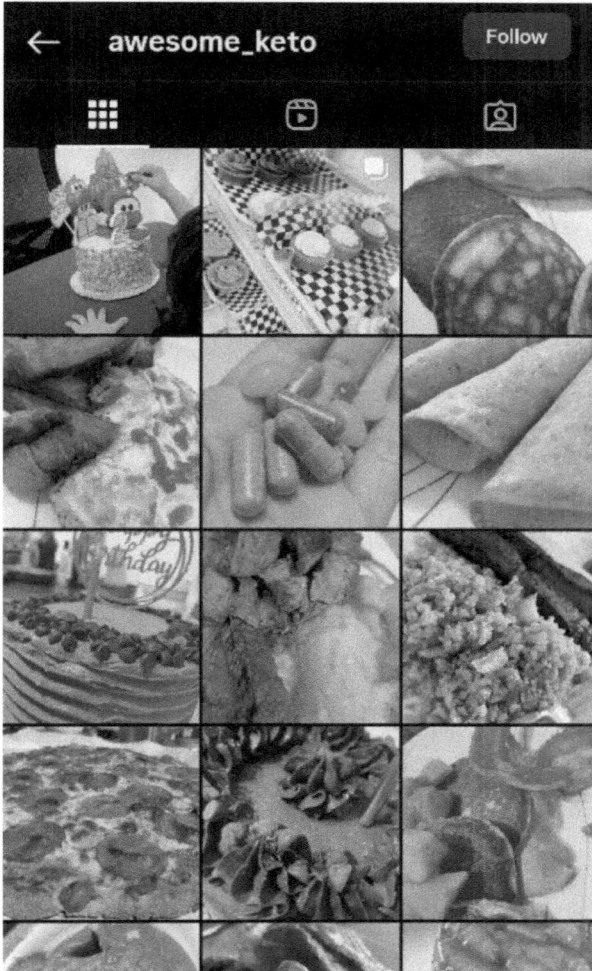

Fig. 4: Inspired by my health journey, my wife and I created a page to share Ketogenic recipes, products, and literature.

6

REINFORCEMENT LEARNING

Living the New Plan

"Discipline yourself, and others won't need to." - Epictetus

Most diets fail because they're neither adaptable nor sustainable, focusing on short-term aesthetic improvement. But what I'd created wasn't just a diet; it was a **dynamic feedback** system that responded to my body's **unique** needs. These tools were working together to fine-tune not just what I ate but also my habits, routines, and entire lifestyle. **They chronicled how I lived**.

And the longer I ran the protocol, the clearer things became. My body didn't just tolerate this way of eating and living; it **thrived** on it.

Gone were the mood crashes, the afternoon slumps, and the unpredictable gut issues that had plagued me for so long. I wasn't continually thinking about food or snacking to "balance my blood sugar". Constant caffeine was no longer a requirement for me to feel awake. I was nourished and thriving, not just managing to get by.

But I knew better than to coast on autopilot.

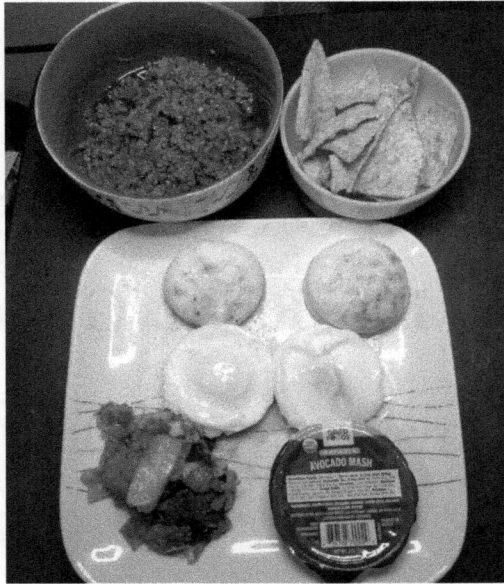

Fig. 1: A typical high-protein breakfast.

Like any long-running system, this lifestyle required observability. So, I continued to collect data, not obsessively, but purposefully. I'd regularly check my HRV after introducing new foods. I'd correlate sleep disruptions with late meals. I'd test how different stressors affected my recovery.

And when something went wrong? I **rolled back** the change, just like in a software deployment pipeline.

This process of continuous improvement slowly revealed a complete diet that took shape over time. To my surprise, it looked eerily familiar, a version of the Ketogenic diet, which I had previously dismissed as a fad.

6.1   Filling the nutrition gaps

One thing I learned is that modern food is severely **nutrient deficient**. Whether it's due to processing, nutritional and raising methods of animals, mass production needs, pesticides, or regulations, the reality is that today's food **alone**, no matter how well you structure your food intake, will always have nutritional **blind spots**.

As I had debugged my food intake, I moved on to supplements. I used the exact measurement and logging approach for each supplement I added, adjusting the intake based on my body's **feedback** and **research** findings.

I started with a multivitamin as a base and then improved the supplementation stack.

6.1.1   Vitamin D

Researching Vitamin D led me to discover that it's a slow but massive **global** health emergency. [203] Vitamin D deficiency contributes silently to countless chronic illnesses.

The numbers are shocking: nearly **half** the world's population is affected.

- **15.7% is severely deficient** (<30 nmol/L).

- **47.9% is deficient** (<50 nmol/L).

- **76.6% is insufficient** (<75 nmol/L).

So, why are we witnessing such a widespread Vitamin D deficiency? The answer lies in its very nature.

Vitamin D is a **fat-soluble** prohormone. To absorb it effectively, your body needs bioavailable dietary fat. Without sufficient fat, the gut cannot properly **dissolve** Vitamin D, hindering absorption.

Now, things made more sense. The way I (and many people) have been taught to eat is by restricting fats.

I realized that restricting fats causes two problems:

- Leads to vitamin D deficiency

- Vitamin D-rich fatty foods like fish, liver, egg yolks, and full-fat dairy are often avoided

Solving my vitamin D deficiency meant **increasing** my fat intake, which I was already doing.

How important is Vitamin D?

Vitamin D is more than just a vitamin; it's a **prohormone** that the body converts into a steroid hormone, **1,25-dihydroxyvitamin D3** (**calcitriol**). This active form of Vitamin D regulates **gene expression** across multiple organ systems and plays a crucial role in maintaining optimal health.

How much Vitamin D do we need?

The recommended daily intake varies based on age, health status, and other factors. A typical recommendation ranges from **400** to **800 IU** (International Units) per day, with an intake of **2,000 IU** as the safe upper limit for the general public. [204]

However, emerging research suggests that daily supplementation of **2,000 IU** may be a more suitable new baseline for maintaining optimal health in adults. [205] Some studies have even explored daily intakes of up to **15,000 IU**, resulting in serum levels reaching **300 nmol/L** with no evidence of **toxicity** or **adverse effects**. [206]

Based on this research and recommendations for individuals following high-fat, low-carbohydrate diets, I've found success with supplementing **10,000 IU** of Vitamin D3 paired with **100 mcg** of vitamin K2.

6.1.2   Vitamin C

When we think of Vitamin C, most of us associate it with just fighting off colds and flu, often referred to as the "orange juice vitamin". However, this nutrient plays a far more significant role in our overall health than just serving as an immune booster.

When we're under stress, whether emotionally, physically, or because of poor sleep or overtraining, our **adrenal glands** go into **overdrive**. They release **cortisol**, **adrenaline**, and **noradrenaline**, triggering the body's "fight-or-flight" response. [207] [208]

These stress hormones cause a rapid **spike in blood sugar** by instructing the liver to dump stored glucose into the bloodstream. However, that's not all; they also stimulate the production of new glucose through a process known as **gluconeogenesis**. [209]

Cortisol promotes the synthesis of glucose from non-carbohydrate sources, while epinephrine increases glucose availability by breaking down glycogen stores. This rapid increase in blood sugar leads to **oxidative stress**, causing damage to tissues, proteins, and even **DNA**.

This type of wear and tear is equal to that seen in **heart disease** and **accelerated aging**. The consequences of prolonged adrenal stress are far-reaching, affecting the heart and vascular system significantly. [210]

Besides being involved in the immune system, Vitamin C is one of your body's most powerful stress regulators. Vitamin C supplementation acts as a potent protector against **adrenal stress** and **inflammation**. [211]

But here's an important nuance: our body's ability to absorb Vitamin C is **not linear**. As oral intake increases, the gastrointestinal system absorbs less, and the kidneys excrete more. [212] This means that once you exceed about **200 mg** of Vitamin C per day, **absorption and retention decrease**. [213]

Additionally, high doses can cause stomach upset, bloating, or diarrhea due to its **acidity**.

That's where **liposomal** Vitamin C comes in. This form **encapsulates** the vitamin in tiny **fat-like particles**, allowing it to bypass the gut transport system and be absorbed more slowly and efficiently. This results in **higher blood levels** over time without the **digestive side effects**. [214]

Vitamin C is considered to have **low toxicity** and is generally regarded as safe, even when consumed in large quantities. Using liposomal Vitamin C enabled me to exceed the absorption limits and achieve **therapeutic** dosages. [215] [216]

Vitamin C isn't just an immune booster; it's **adrenal armor**. But here's the thing: it's not just about how much Vitamin C you take; it's also about how well your body can use it.

6.1.3 Zinc

As I progressed further into my research on supplementation, zinc emerged as another eye-opening revelation.

You've probably never craved a serving of zinc the way you might crave steak or salt. But your body? It's **begging** for it, every hour of every day. Zinc is no second-rate nutrient; it's a vital component that deserves attention beyond the confines of the cold season.

Here's a surprising truth: zinc acts more like a **hormone than a mineral**. It turns genes on, guides over 300 enzymes, and protects your DNA like a molecular bodyguard. [217]

And when you don't get enough of it? Things fall apart. Your immune function falters, inflammation spirals out of control, and your overall health begins to deteriorate.

Zinc plays a vital role in supporting **immune cells**, including T cells and B cells, as well as regulating the production of **cytokines**. A deficiency can **impair** immune responses, making you more susceptible to infections and prolonged inflammatory states. [218]

Zinc's significance extends beyond immunity; it's essential for **growth**, **development**, and **reproduction**. Adequate zinc levels are vital during periods of rapid growth, such as infancy, adolescence, and pregnancy. Zinc deficiency during these critical periods can lead to **growth retardation**, **delayed sexual maturation**, and complications during **pregnancy and childbirth**. [219]

Zinc has a significant role in neurological function. It acts as a **neuromodulator**, playing a role in synaptic transmission. Altered zinc levels have been linked to mood disorders, cognitive impairments, and an increased risk of **neurodegenerative diseases**. [220]

One of the most impressive aspects of zinc is its antioxidant properties. Zinc contributes to the body's antioxidant defense system by **stabilizing cell membranes** and **neutralizing free radicals**. This function is crucial in preventing cellular damage and reducing the risk of chronic diseases. [221] [222]

Interestingly, **pairing** zinc with animal protein can enhance absorption. [223] [224] By combining these two essential nutrients, I was able to unlock even greater benefits from my diet.

Now, the bad news.

Zinc deficiency affects a staggering number of people. Estimates range from **17% to 20%** of the global population, which translates to over **1.5 billion** individuals. [225]

The good news?

Zinc is an **inexpensive, widely available**, and **highly effective** nutrient when taken in proper amounts.

6.1.4 Creatine

I used to think creatine was just for gym goers.

When I first started taking creatine, it was primarily to support my exercise routine. However, what caught my attention were the studies that linked creatine to improved **artery health, better blood sugar control**, and even **stroke prevention**. These benefits of creatine blew my mind! I had no idea about its potential impact on cardiovascular health.

One study showed that older adults who took creatine for just four weeks experienced significant improvements in **endothelial function** (this word would become very significant to me later on); essentially, their arteries began to work like those of younger individuals. And that kind of improvement? It's tied to a lower risk of **heart attacks** and **strokes**. [226]

But that's not all; the same study found:

- **Improved blood flow** to small vessels

- **Lower fasting glucose** levels and **triglycerides**

- **No spike in oxidative stress**, showing that creatine doesn't overburden the system

Another trial revealed that older men who took creatine experienced **reduced arterial stiffness** and even saw a drop in their **blood pressure** of 8 points. Although this blood pressure reduction wasn't statistically significant, it was directionally promising. [227]

It stunned me to discover that creatine isn't just a supplement for athletes; it's a vital molecule in cellular energy processes, primarily within muscles and especially in the heart. Some **heart conditions** are associated with **low creatine** levels or impaired creatine metabolism. [228]

We get most of our creatine from **red meat** and **fish**. This fact was another validation for my decision to base my diet on animal protein.

This knowledge has given me a new perspective on creatine: like animal fat and protein, it's often **misunderstood**, possibly even **stigmatized**, but **absolutely essential**.

Creatine isn't merely for athletes. It's for anyone who has a heart.

6.1.5 Salt

At first glance, it might seem illogical to follow a low-carbohydrate diet when struggling with heart health issues. After all, low-carbohydrate diets often lead to **excessive fluid loss**. And if you're prone to hypotension, wouldn't that make it an even greater concern? "Common sense" would suggest steering clear of low-carbohydrate diets altogether.

But my experience and data told a different story. By **combining** a high-sodium diet with a hypocaloric diet and nutrient-dense foods, I found that the body's fluid levels remained stable, a state known as **euvolemia** rather than **hypovolemia**. Instead of making it worse, this **improved** my postural hypotension.

But how did I know this? The answer lies in real-time feedback from my electrocardiogram (ECG) readings. While adjusting my salt intake, I noticed that as I stood up, my heart stress was significantly **reduced**, which meant that my vascular system was regulating blood pressure much more effectively. My heart no longer had to work overtime to compensate for the dip in blood pressure.

With salt intake advice, I again noticed the same mindset of treating health conditions with a single nutritional approach, which is not only oversimplified but also misguided. The body is a complex system, and problems in one organ are commonly identified as pathologies when they are often symptoms of underlying issues elsewhere.

Since studies have shown that low sodium intake alone can improve hypertension, [229] one might rationalize that high sodium intake would also improve postural hypotension; yet, this is not the case. [230]

A hypocaloric diet supports **aldosterone regulation** without worsening **cardiometabolic markers**. [231] Aldosterone is a mineralocorticoid hormone produced by the adrenal glands that regulates sodium and water retention and influences blood pressure.

While there may not be direct studies on the combined effects of high sodium intake and ketogenic diets on kidney sodium handling, it appears that **together**, they have a synergistic effect on my health, improving kidney **sodium handling**, restoring **isotonic balance**, and helping to prevent both **hypovolemia** and **orthostatic hypotension**.

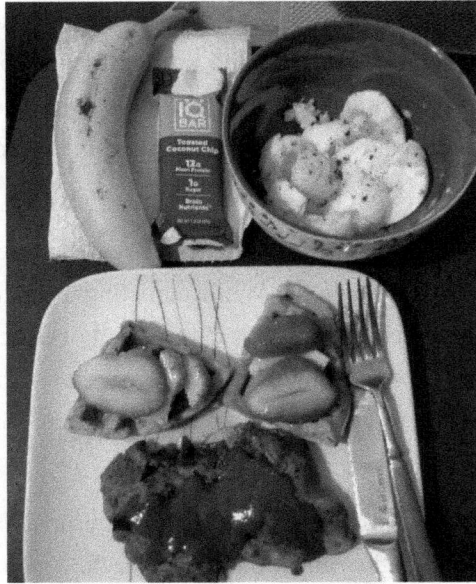

Fig. 2: A typical high-protein brunch.

6.2   Understanding fats

Since increasing my intake of dietary fats had such a positive impact on my well-being, I began researching how fats function in the body.

For years, fats had been my nemesis, an enemy that I thought simply accumulated under the skin or floated aimlessly through the bloodstream. Boy, was I wrong!

The human body doesn't operate like a free-for-all, where substances can drift haphazardly through our systems. Instead, it carefully manages everything, and fat storage is no exception.

A specialized group of cells called **adipocytes** is responsible for managing fats in the body. [232] These cells not only store, release, and transport lipids but also tightly control energy distribution and structural fat functions.

Unlike carbohydrates, fats play multiple critical roles in the body. They

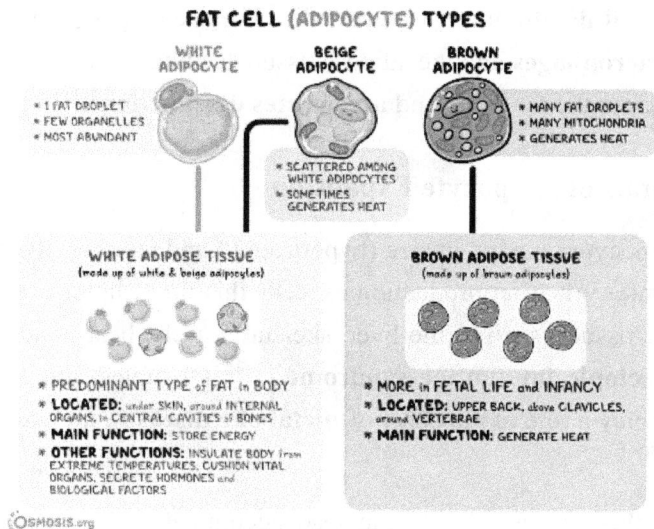

Fig. 3: Types of adipocytes.

provide energy, aid in hormone synthesis, support the absorption of essential vitamins and minerals, and are necessary for healthy **cell membranes** and **signaling pathways**.

Carbohydrates, on the other hand, are primarily just a source of energy.

Besides their unbalanced benefits when compared to fats, high-carbohydrate diets raise **insulin levels**, **increase hunger**, **reduce energy expenditure**, and trigger hormonal changes that promote **accelerated fat storage**. [233]

As demand for fat accumulation increases, the body responds by producing more adipocytes. When existing fat cells reach their capacity, precursor cells known as preadipocytes undergo a process called **adipogenesis**, during which they divide and mature into new fat cells. This process can lead to **adipocyte hyperplasia**. [234] Adipocyte hyperplasia, in turn, contributes to **obesity** and **metabolic diseases**.

But that's not the end of it. When adipocytes become over-engorged with lipids, pathological changes occur, including **cellular senescence**, accelerated **cell death**, and even **necrosis**. These changes attract immune cells and **macrophages** into the adipose tissue, leading to inflammation that further damages the fat tissue and **accelerates dysfunction**. [235]

6.2.1 Limits of Adipocyte Expansion

Even as adipocytes expand in size (hypertrophy) and number (hyperplasia), there's a limit. When fat production exceeds this limit, lipids are stored in non-adipose tissues, such as the liver, skeletal muscle, heart, and pancreas, leading to **ectopic fat storage syndrome**. [236] Disrupted adipogenesis is believed to play a role in the onset of **metabolic diseases**, including **type 2 diabetes**. [237]

As part of this process, lipids can also accumulate in the bloodstream, contributing to the onset of **hyperlipidemia**. Hyperlipidemia, in turn, triggers a buildup of inflammatory **leukocytes in arterial walls**, which contributes to the development of **atherosclerosis**. [238]

Excess fat that is redirected to the liver leads to lipid overload, attracting inflammatory monocytes that transform into macrophages. Inflammatory T-cell populations, such as Th1 cells, cytotoxic T lymphocytes (CTLs), and Th17 cells, also infiltrate the liver, triggering a **cascade of inflammation** that further compromises the liver's function. [239]

As I progressed further into the intricate mechanisms of lipid handling, I began to appreciate the complex interplay between this process and the immune system. These findings validated my data and solidified my commitment to a low-carbohydrate diet.

The adverse effects of dietary carbohydrates, as opposed to dietary fat, destroyed all my preconceived notions of energy consumption and expenditure.

This new understanding even made me question long-held beliefs about exercise, which became the next area I explored.

6.3 Workouts

For two decades, I dedicated myself to martial arts training, convinced I knew everything there was to know about exercise, training, and weightlifting.

But I continued rebuilding from first principles, only to be astonished by how much conventional wisdom on fitness prioritized **aesthetics** over actual **health benefits**.

The notion of "fitness" has become a euphemism for poor health in disguise. Behind the gleaming facade, many people are hiding a darker truth: their bodies may be buffed up on the **outside**, but their health is still suffering on the **inside**.

6.3.1 Dangerous extremes

With fresh eyes, I realized that many fitness recommendations were addressing **emotional** and **psychological** problems under the guise of improving health. Studies have linked **muscle dysmorphia** (MD) in bodybuilders to anxiety, social physique anxiety, depression, neuroticism, and perfectionism, negatively affecting **self-concept** and **self-esteem**. [240]

Modern fitness has a puzzling twist: despite its reputation for physical excellence, competitive bodybuilders are more likely to suffer from **health problems** and **higher mortality rates** than the general public. [241]

High-intensity training programs, such as CrossFit, don't fare much better either. CrossFit has been linked in the literature to injury rates as high as **20%**. [242] Besides its high injury rate, CrossFit training may result in multiple adverse health outcomes, including **exertional rhabdomyolysis**. Rhabdomyolysis is a condition in which damaged skeletal muscle tissue breaks down rapidly, releasing intracellular contents, such as myoglobin, into the bloodstream.

Exertional rhabdomyolysis can result in **acute kidney injury** (AKI). In severe cases, the kidney impairment meets the RIFLE criteria (Risk, Injury,

Failure, Loss, End-stage renal disease) to classify it as **end-stage renal disease**. [243] [244] [245] Knowledge of this consequence of CrossFit is not rare or new. [246]

I was surprised to learn that among CrossFit circles, rhabdomyolysis has been turned into a caricature named "Pukie the Clown", also known as "Uncle Rhabdo", named after the condition from which he is suffering. [247]

As I dug deeper, I realized how many fitness programs go to incredible lengths to craft **elaborate routines** and sell you the **latest equipment** but rarely outline the specific, **research-backed health benefits** of their programs.

Likewise, I started to question the obsession with **muscle group isolation**. I've trained that way before, making significant gains only to become injured because I hadn't prioritized training the stabilizer muscles with the same intensity.

My goal was no longer just hypertrophy but **neural adaptation**, **usable strength**, and **neuromuscular improvements**. [248] This new goal led me to explore alternative training philosophies, where I stumbled upon **Mike Mentzer's High-Intensity Training** (HIT). This method emphasizes high-intensity, low-volume training and strict technique to maximize muscle growth with minimal time commitment. [249]

I was intrigued by the idea of "training to failure", performing a single set of an exercise until **absolute exhaustion** instead of multiple sets. Mentzer emphasized that once a muscle is fatigued, additional sets are **unnecessary** and potentially **counterproductive**.

He also recommended long rest periods of **4 to 7** days between sessions to maximize muscle rebuilding as opposed to the common practice of interleaving workout days with rest days.

Another interesting aspect of the Mentzer method was the idea that holding the weight until failure could be an effective alternative to a set of repetitions. Emphasizing leveraging the muscle's **sustained** and **negative strengths** during the exercise.

While hypertrophy was no longer my primary goal, his training philosophy had appeal as a means to avoid training blind spots and increase workout efficiency.

6.3.2   Old school, new school

As I learned more about the Mentzer Method further, my curiosity was piqued, leading me down a rabbit hole of exploration into older training regimens and philosophies that had shaped the world of bodybuilding. This journey ultimately landed me on the concept of "Bodybuilding Eras", a framework that breaks down the history of the sport into distinct periods: the **Bronze Era** (1900-1930), the **Silver Era** (1930-1960), and the **Golden Era** (1960-1990).

The further I ventured back in time, the more striking it became that these pioneering bodybuilders lived in a world **without** modern supplements, anabolic steroids, or cutting-edge nutrition products. Instead, they relied on **unprocessed protein, high-fat diets**, and **low-carbohydrate intake**, often pushing their bodies into a state of **ketosis**. Old-school bodybuilders didn't just talk about ketosis; it was a natural byproduct of their diets.

Interestingly, research indicates that elite athletes who adhered to older bodybuilding philosophies had a striking **reversal** in the sport's relationship with longevity. [250]

As I experimented with these methods myself, I discovered that some adaptations had a profound effect on my health conditions, particularly **orthostatic intolerance.** [251] By focusing on building strong leg muscle tone, I was able to improve the regulation of my blood pressure and even my circulatory function.   This finding challenged my previous understanding of the importance of legs in overall health.

Another win to combat hypotension!

The truth is that our legs are more than just passive supports. They're **active pumps**, almost like a "second heart". When you walk, stand up, flex, or even just tense your calves and thighs, you help push blood back up to your heart and brain. This phenomenon is known as the **muscle pump mechanism**, a crucial aspect of maintaining stable blood pressure, particularly for those struggling with hypotension. [252]

Studies have shown that lower limb resistance training can have a direct impact on **orthostatic tolerance**. [253] Moreover, research has shown that leg exercises enhance **baroreflex sensitivity**, [254] a crucial factor in maintaining stable blood pressure. Through low-resistance training, individuals can improve vascular tone and autonomic regulation. Both are essential for stable blood pressure. [255]

6.3.3   Rebooting my fitness routine

Bottom line?

I embarked on a research-driven journey to overhaul my approach to exercise. If your legs are weak, your circulation suffers. If your circulation suffers, **everything** suffers as a result.

And so, I researched, made changes, tested, and measured the results. Now, in my workouts, I focus on the following:

- **Mobility**. Paying attention to the hips, calves, and ankles.

- Aim to **tire** and **fail** the muscle, not just pursue the **burn** and the **pump**.

- Train for health, **not looks**.

- **Limit** my sessions to no more than 40 minutes, 3 times a week.

- Focus on training that mimics **natural** movements.

- Cover not just **brute force** but flexibility, agility, sustained strength, and stamina.

This hybrid system blends elements of **high-intensity interval training** (HIIT), **calisthenics, cardio, plyometrics, rotational exercises**, and **yoga**.

By doing so, I've managed to break free from the cult of fitness for aesthetics that often dominates our culture. Instead, I focus on **function** and **longevity**, the actual keys to optimal health.

That's how I rebuilt the pump system I didn't know I had. That's how I **stood back up**, literally and metaphorically.

6.4 The final piece

Like other misconceptions that stem from oversimplification and compartmentalization of health and biology, I always thought blood vessels were simple tubes with some muscle, just that. A bit of research revealed that blood vessels are far more complex and sophisticated than I had ever imagined.

As I delved deeper into researching vasoconstriction and baroreceptors to understand my hypotension, I stumbled upon the **endothelial glycocalyx**. The more I read about this structure, the more I realized I'd struck gold! I was on the cusp of a **major breakthrough** in understanding my hypotension.

The endothelial glycocalyx was once thought to be a passive physical barrier. However, it's now recognized as a **multifunctional** and **dynamic** structure that's critically important for various vascular processes, including **vascular permeability, inflammation, thrombosis, mechanotransduction**, and **cytokine signaling**. [256]

As a sensor of blood flow, the glycocalyx helps the endothelium (the lining of blood vessels) respond to **shear stress**, the friction caused by blood flowing through vessels.

However, here's the fascinating part: the glycocalyx is not just a passive sensor of stress; it **actively** responds by releasing **nitric oxide** (NO), which

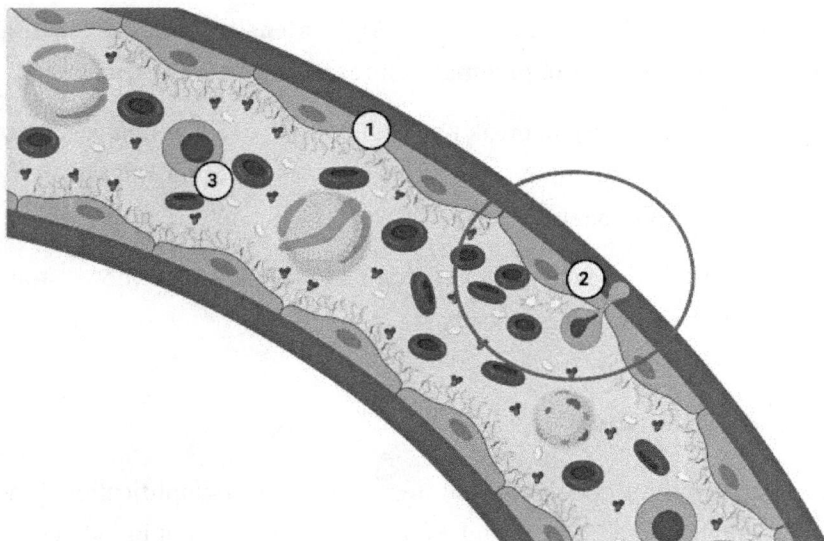

Fig. 4: Blood vessel diagram showing glycocalyx as object number 1.

causes changes in vessel diameter to ensure proper tissue perfusion. This process of **mechanotransduction** refers to the cellular mechanisms that convert physical forces into biochemical signals and adapt responses accordingly.

The influence of shear stress on endothelial morphology and function has been well documented, but it has **only recently** begun to be attributed to the glycocalyx. [257] [258]

6.4.1 Impaired glycocalyx

The link between endothelial dysfunction, cardiovascular, and metabolic diseases is well-established. [259] However, the primary root cause of this dysfunction appears to be a **compromised glycocalyx**.

Through an interplay of mechanisms, glycocalyx injury can trigger abnormal **vasoconstriction** and **vasodilation**. [260] [261] [262]

Let's look closer at the scenarios that lead to vasoconstriction:

- Reduced endothelial response to shear stress.

- Impaired nitric oxide (NO) production.

- The binding of leukocytes and platelets to exposed endothelial cells. This triggers endothelial inflammation, impairs blood flow, and induces vasoconstriction through endothelin-1.

Now, for the scenarios that result in vasodilation:

- Vascular hyper-permeability leading to fluid leakage from blood vessels and hypotension.

- Excessive nitric oxide (NO) production in response to inflammatory cytokines.

In my case, **chronic inflammation** and the **constant release** of inflammatory mediators, cytokines, and prostaglandins drove **excessive nitric oxide** (NO) production. Lifelong damage to the glycocalyx had plunged me into a persistent state of **decreased vascular tone** and **systemic vascular vasodilation**.

The integrity of the glycocalyx is inextricably linked to blood flow. Healthy shear stress from normal blood flow maintains its thickness and function. Conversely, **reduced shear stress**, caused by vasoconstriction or impaired blood flow, leads to **degradation** of the glycocalyx. This link establishes a feedback loop in which blood flow and glycocalyx integrity are **mutually reinforcing**. [257]

To make matters worse, the glycocalyx plays a fundamental role in the formation, stabilization, and maturation of blood vessels. Damage or dysfunction of this delicate structure can compromise vascular integrity, leading to **impaired blood vessel development**. [263] [264]

This is the worst "chicken and egg" problem I've ever seen!

6.4.2 The main culprit

Of all the potential solutions to prevent glycocalyx damage, the simplest, although not necessarily the easiest, is to **reduce high blood sugar** levels.

High sugar levels, particularly within the context of diabetes and hyperglycemia, can inflict significant harm on the glycocalyx through a process called **lipotoxicity**. [265] However, it's not just about elevated glucose; a high-carbohydrate diet alone can also trigger this degradation.

Advanced glycation end products (AGEs) form when sugars, particularly glucose and fructose, bind non-enzymatically to proteins and lipids. This glycation process is accelerated when:

- **Blood glucose levels are elevated**, as seen with high-carbohydrate diets or poorly controlled diabetes.

- **Fructose intake is high** (think high-fructose corn syrup), which generates AGEs at a faster rate than glucose.

- **There's oxidative stress**, frequently heightened in high-carb, high-glycemic diets.

A high carbohydrate intake, especially refined or high-glycemic-index carbohydrates, significantly increases endogenous AGE formation.

It's crucial to understand that AGEs aren't just **passive indicators** of glycocalyx damage; they **actively contribute** to its degradation. [266] [267] In addition to AGEs, even just high glucose levels themselves can trigger this destructive process. [268]

6.4.3 Solution

Here comes the good news. Finally!

The glycocalyx **can regenerate**. [269]

All I needed to do was lower AGE production. That was surprisingly easy, as ketogenic or low-carbohydrate diets resulted in:

- **Lower blood glucose and insulin levels**, thereby reducing the raw materials needed for AGE formation.

- **Lower oxidative stress** due to improved mitochondrial function and reduced glucose-related **reactive oxygen species** (ROS).

- **Reduced inflammation**, which slows AGE accumulation and damage.

Time and again, a diet low in carbohydrates, high in fat, and rich in animal proteins, combined with complete supplementation, has emerged as the **most effective** approach to help regenerate and protect the glycocalyx. [270]

I'd finally found the last piece of my health puzzle. I'd completed the picture of my symptom and conditions stack.

The root cause has **always** been damage to the **glycocalyx** resulting from a lifetime of **high dietary carbohydrates** combined with **low** nutritional **fats** and animal **protein**.

A bad diet since early in life kept my glycocalyx in a degraded state. Without a properly functioning glycocalyx, my arteries, particularly those in my legs, suffered developmental issues, exhibiting severe deficiencies in vascular tone, baroreception, and the vasoconstriction reflex. This vascular deficiency, in turn, led to chronic hypotension. The almost constant compensatory tachycardia followed, resulting in low-grade chronic myocardial infarction. The myocardial injury, finally, triggered nerve sprouting. And we arrive at the starting point: supraventricular tachycardia (SVT) and all my other heart issues.

Diet was the catalyst, then compounded by the persistent hypotension and impaired blood flow, kept the glycocalyx in a compromised state, creating a **self-feeding cycle of chronic illness**.

The journey was long and winding, but I finally cracked the code to my health!

I inverted the proportions of my diet, added targeted supplementation, and implemented a restorative exercise program. These changes quickly promoted the regeneration of my glycocalyx, and I experienced a positive ripple effect, ultimately resulting in a calm and proper heart rhythm and function.

6.5 The results

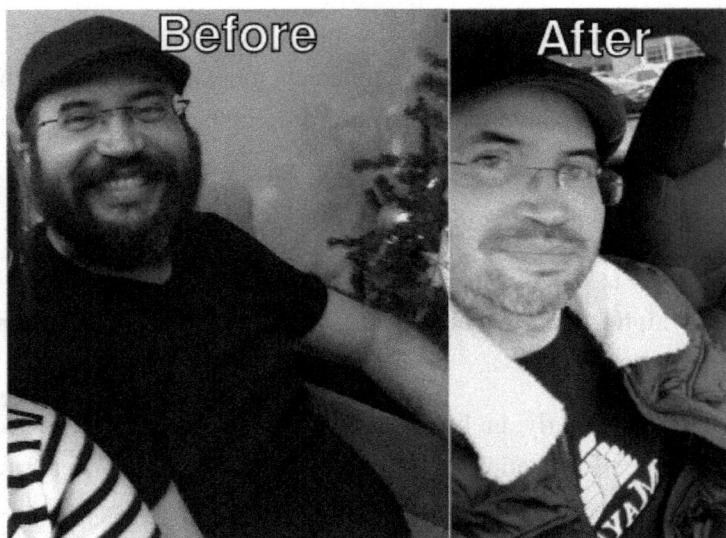

Fig. 5: Before and after comparison. Three years and ten days later (December 2016, January 2020).

Recording and measuring everything became my default mode. The positive effects became not just self-evident but painfully obvious to my shame.

This wasn't biohacking in the trendy sense; it was **systemic stability engineering**. I treated my body the way I treat mission-critical software: with respect for complexity and a commitment to uptime.

That meant logging, profiling, researching, experimenting, reviewing, correlating, and repeating ad nauseam.

Over time, the system required fewer interventions. My baseline had shifted.

My "default state" was now **healthy**.

I was no longer dependent on medications; I stopped needing **propafenone** and **aspirin** to control my arrhythmia in 2018. Also gone were their side effects and interactions. [271] [272] [273] [274] [275] [276]

I also dropped NSAIDs and corticosteroids, along with other medications.

No flare-ups. No mystery symptoms. Just solid, sustainable wellbeing.

That didn't mean I stopped learning. I continued to read new research, compare nutrient profiles, and test fasting windows. But I no longer chased novelty. I chased **resilience**.

And it held.

Slowly but surely, I fine-tuned my diet. I ended up with a **modified Ketogenic diet** that favors **high amounts of animal protein** (mainly from red meat), **less dietary fat** than the standard ketogenic diet, and dictates **very few carbohydrates**, only from natural, low-glycemic sources, such as **berries** and a **few carefully** selected vegetables.

Paired with a supplement protocol that focused on metabolic, regenerative, immune, and cardiovascular health, I finally had my ideal diet.

Together with my new workout regimen, I had finally developed my **wellness protocol**.

From 2018 onward, I didn't just survive; I optimized. I gained lean muscle without inflammation. My sleep improved without pills. My mind stayed sharp through long development sprints. And I could predict, with stunning accuracy, how a meal would affect my physiology.

The transition from Orthostatic Hypotension (OH) (or poor) to Initial Orthostatic Hypotension (IOH) (or normal) is not well-documented as a defined clinical pathway in the medical literature. Yet, I experienced it firsthand in my own body. Several aspects of my health and biomarkers were **regressing**, exhibiting a "reverse aging" pattern, indicating that they were moving towards values associated with younger individuals. I wasn't getting younger, but the pace of age-related changes was slowing; I was **aging slower**.

The best of all? This lifestyle didn't feel restrictive. It felt empowering. I wasn't at the mercy of cravings, mood swings, or marketing. I wasn't dependent on expert opinions. I had built a relationship with my body based on **data**, **trust**, and **iteration**.

I didn't follow a plan; I **engineered** one.

And in 2025, when **everything** was on the line again, I'd learn just how much that mattered.

7

SECOND TEST

The 2025 Emergency Surgery

"It's not what happens to you, but how you react to it, that matters." - Epictetus

You never truly know how robust your system is until it's pushed to its absolute limits under a failure scenario.

It happened in 2025. Six hours. That's all it took to rip me from a typical day and plunge me into a full-blown medical emergency.

7.1   The worst pain ever

It began on a Sunday with a simple errand: a four-hour road trip, and it couldn't be canceled. As I pulled out the door, a dull ache settled in the center of my stomach. Faint at first, a whisper of discomfort, so I decided to push through; the errand was also time-sensitive.

But while driving down the highway, the pain slowly intensified. Along with the increased pain, my abdomen was also swelling, together with a strange feeling of pressure. The sense of pressure was not outward but **inward**, as if something was pressing down on my **navel** and my **breastbone**. Initially, I blamed it on something I'd eaten for breakfast, a minor digestive hiccup.

After completing my task at the destination, I stopped at a nearby coffee shop. "Maybe a macchiato would soothe the stomach", I thought. I also used the ambiance to get some work done, a mental distraction from the growing discomfort.

Forty minutes later, the ache had solidified into a sharp, undeniable pain. It was hard to ignore. I decided it was time to start the long trip back.

> *I'd driven myself to the hospital with a fractured forearm and endured tournaments with cracked ribs. Yet, this pain was different. On a scale of 1 to 10, it was now a **15**.*

As I got into my car, I was struck by how swollen my belly had become. I had to loosen the belt just to sit comfortably. *"Haven't had food poisoning this bad in years"*, I thought. While backing out, the pain **exploded**. It was so intense, so sudden, that I had the sensation that I was going to faint. This pain wasn't food poisoning. This pain was something else. **Something bad**.

The pain was also spreading, starting in my belly, then **radiating** outwards, encompassing my entire abdomen, even my chest and rib cage. I was still an hour and a half away, and the pain was **escalating**, accelerating with terrifying speed. I needed to get back home, and fast.

I'd read about heart attacks; some cause pain that is felt in the stomach. Was something grave happening internally, stressing my heart and causing chest pain? Or was I having a heart attack, and the stomach pain was just a symptom?

Halfway back, I called my wife to get her up to speed. Still, I insisted it could be nothing. I was clinging to denial, not wanting to worry her unnecessarily. Desperately, I was trying to avoid repeating the events and uncertainty we'd endured before in 2016. But even as I spoke, it became brutally clear: this pain wasn't ordinary; it was a **warning** bell ringing loud and clear.

My delay in drinking coffee, compounded by the ever-present Puerto Rican traffic jams, stretched the trip back to two and a half hours.

I'm no stranger to pain and have learned to tolerate it well. Years of suffering from hypocalcemia had resulted in frequently fractured bones. I'd driven myself to the hospital with a fractured forearm and endured tournaments with cracked ribs. Yet, this pain was different. On a scale of 1 to 10, it was now a **15**.

When I got home, my wife had some tea waiting for me. Since dropping all antacids and stomach medication, on the rare occasions when I got an upset stomach, star anise tea always worked. Not this time. There was barely any improvement. Later, she remarked that my belly was so swollen that the skin looked "*shiny*".

We started making preparations to go to the ER, just in case. I tried lying down and resting, hoping it would subside. Twenty minutes later, I couldn't **stand it anymore**.

When I told my wife I agreed to be driven to the hospital because I couldn't withstand the pain, she knew it was a big deal.

7.2 The ER, my old friend

The drive to the ER felt like an eternity. Every bump, every vibration of the road spiked the pain.

As soon as we arrived, I notified the staff about the chest pain and also mentioned my history of heart conditions, triggering a rapid response protocol. Within minutes, they were taking vital signs, drawing blood, and starting the first of several EKGs.

The results were unsettling. Besides the sheer intensity of the pain, my heart enzymes, specifically Troponin, were elevated, something now rare for me. Those levels very likely meant **sudden** and **severe** myocardial injury or **sepsis**. [277] A chest X-ray, followed by another EKG and an echocardiogram, confirmed the grim possibility: there had been a **heart attack**, but not a classic one.

The pain and the inflammation were all complementing a cascade of physiological responses and an increased cardiac workload. This created a supply-and-demand mismatch in the coronary circulation. Which, in turn, was causing a sudden myocardial injury and elevated Troponin levels.

This is called a temporary **Type 2 myocardial infarction** (MI). A serious condition, indeed, but not as immediately life-threatening as a **Type 1 MI**, the one caused by a complete blockage of a coronary artery. Given the clinical context, it was expected. It was a symptom of the undetermined but broader systemic illness **raging** through me.

Next, the ER staff addressed the abdominal pain. A sonogram revealed a major amount of intestinal swelling. A CT scan was ordered to provide more detailed information and to map the extent of the problem.

7.3   Unexpected diagnostic

While related to the digestive system, it wasn't a problem with my stomach. The CT scan result was conclusive: **advanced appendicitis**.

The appendix had to be removed as soon as possible, "*a routine procedure*", they assured me: laparoscopic surgery, a quick recovery. However, the Troponin levels needed to decrease first.

I was admitted, immediately administered **intravenous** (IV) antibiotics, and authorized a dose of morphine every four hours, a temporary relief from the relentless pain. To prepare for surgery, I couldn't eat anything, **not even drink water**.

The Troponin levels and the swelling took **four days** to subside. Four days of nothing. A complete, deliberate fast. Fortunately, prolonged fasting was nothing new to me, a consequence of the things I've learned and the strategies I've implemented.

7.4 Surgery

The eagerly awaited day finally arrived.

I was prepped and wheeled in early. The surgeon had block-booked the operating room for the day and prioritized me due to my emergency state. [278] I vaguely remember the staff introducing themselves. Then, I felt the cold sting of the anesthesia in my left arm's vein. Shortly after, I slipped into the darkness.

When I woke, the first thing that slammed into me was the intense, throbbing pain all over my abdomen. It felt as if my insides had been yanked out, tossed around like a deck of cards, and then shoved back in.

Barely conscious, still tethered to the operating room, I managed to croak out to the nurse, "*It hurts a lot*". She immediately administered morphine, and fleeting warmth spread through my body. It didn't quite reach the core of the pain.

Someone from surgery wheeled me back to my room. All I remember were the slow, hypnotic transiting lights of the hospital room ceilings. Back in the room, I faced a new challenge: transferring from the operating room gurney to my bed. I had to lie on my side while the nurse slid a board and a blanket under my back.

Something so utterly unremarkable in the past was now a gargantuan maneuver, demanding Olympian strength and offering only infernal pain in return. I felt my organs shifting freely within my abdomen. It was a disconcerting sensation for what should have been a straightforward procedure. With a few tugs of the blanket, I was finally back in my bed. I slid again into nothing.

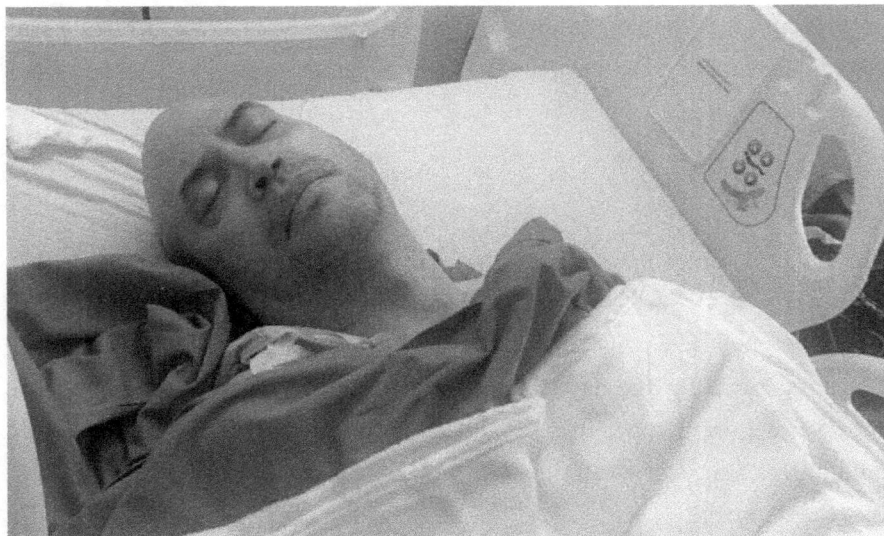

Fig. 1: Just out of surgery.

7.5 Not-so-routine surgery

The surgeon came to see me later that afternoon. He explained that he'd started a routine laparoscopic appendectomy, looked inside, and immediately had to abandon the original plan.

The appendix had twisted backward, stubbornly out of reach. He needed to perform a full laparotomy, an emergency abdominal surgery. The surgeon did so because I was experiencing peritonitis. My appendix had become gangrenous and ruptured. The rupture was, fortunately, stable and not progressing. However, the surrounding tissue had become necrotic. The situation demanded immediate, meticulous care and decisive action. Speed was of the essence to prevent full-on sepsis from occurring.

Due to the necrosis, my cecum, the beginning of the ascending colon, and the last section of the small intestine also needed to be removed. It is a process called an **Ileo-Caecal resection**. [279]

Then, after the removal, the small intestine had to be painstakingly

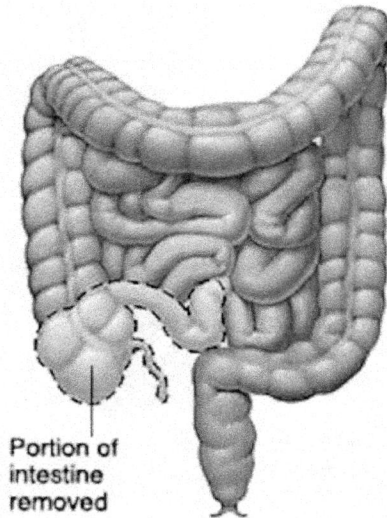

Fig. 2: Removal of the Appendix, Cecum, and Ileocecal valve.

reattached to the large intestine via a procedure called **anastomosis**. [280]

For most people, this would mean a risk of anastomotic leakage, a painful recovery, and months of rehabilitation. But the surgeon reassured me my situation wasn't typical.

I wasn't like any of his other patients.

7.6 My surgical profile

I can still recall the surgeon's face, a genuine expression of amazement, as he recounted my **pain tolerance**, my elevated post-operative **awareness** after just a few hours, and the results of my **blood work**. He was particularly astounded by my **albumin level**.

This wasn't an accident; **my body had been prepared**.

The surgeon meticulously walked me through my profile:

- **Albumin level:** 5.0 g/dL.

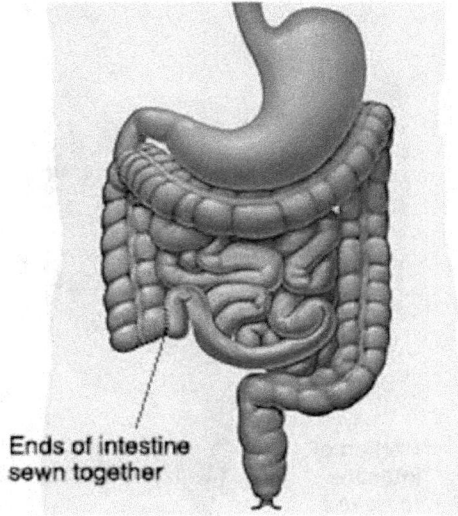

Fig. 3: Reattachment of the Ileum to the large intestine.

- **Inflammatory markers:** Remarkably low.

- **Electrolyte balance:** Stable.

- **Microbiome response to antibiotics:** Astonishingly resilient. No gut issues, no signs of dysbiosis.

- **Pain tolerance:** Simply off the charts.

Word quickly got out. When visiting for checkups, doctors and nurses would consistently ask me the same question: *"What are you doing differently?"*

I'd simply reply, *"I eat exactly what my body wants, not what the food pyramid dictates"*.

7.7   Recovery

My recovery was lightning-fast. Twenty-four hours after surgery, I was ingesting liquefied food and bone broth.

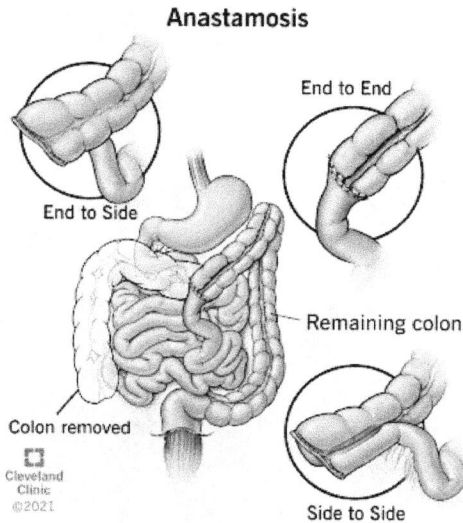

Anastamosis

End to Side

End to End

Remaining colon

Colon removed

Cleveland Clinic ©2021

Side to Side

Fig. 4: Anastomosis types.

The next day? I was up on my own, texting with my family and snapping selfies on my feet, a blatant, joyful proof of my progress.

By the third day, I was eating scrambled eggs and mashed food, bathing on my own, and taking care of myself with surprising ease. I didn't need morphine for the pain anymore. I was trimming my hair and shaving as usual. This felt less like recovery from an operation and more like a hotel stay.

The next day, the surgeon arrived with a big smile on his face, having witnessed my rapid progress. *"Are you ready to move to solid food?"* he asked.

That day, I **devoured** a succulent roast beef for dinner.

Fueled by solid food and a curated regimen of supplements, protein shakes, protein bars, bone broth, cheeses, and ham snacks, I turbo-boosted my recovery even further. Five days after my surgery, I was ready to be discharged.

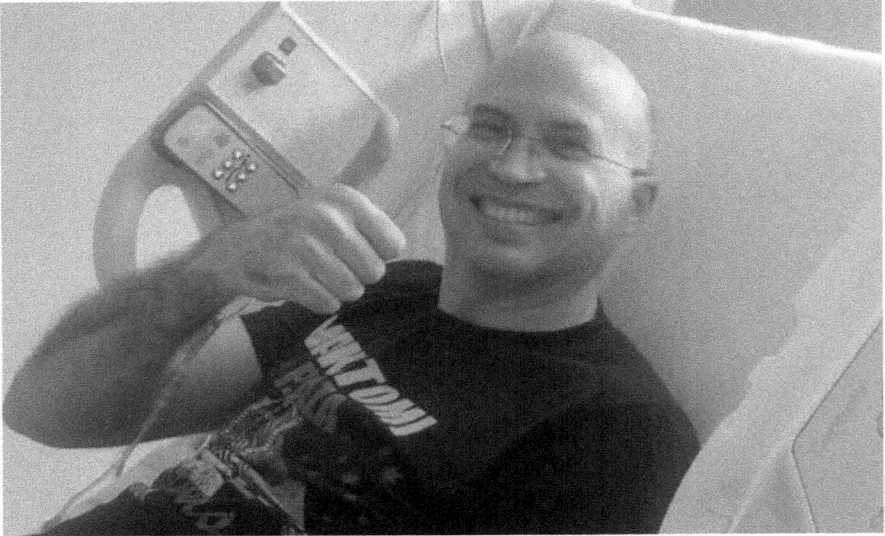

Fig. 5: Excellent recovery in just 4 days.

The only reason I remained in the hospital for two more days was because my youngest son had the flu. If I were to catch it, the persistent coughing or sneezing could very well have led to a hernia.

Two extra days of rest? What better use of them than to start outlining **this very book**?

7.8   A true holistic approach

When asked about my "method", it was challenging to convey all the extensive research and resolution I'd undertaken to address my past conditions. So, I simply summarized it as better food, a customized diet. But it was **far more** than that.

The word "holistic" had been so overused it had lost its true meaning. Holistic doesn't just mean considering more than one body system. Holistic means "the whole". It must consider all aspects of the situation, not just all **the parts of the subject** but also the **processes** and the **environment**.

I've been engaged in truly holistic iterative design on myself. I've been taking into account not just the subject, me, but also all the other aspects surrounding and affecting me. Because of this, I wasn't guessing. I'd engineered my biology to be anti-fragile.

Even in the **worst-case** scenario of a ruptured organ, emergency surgery, and delayed intervention, my healing was rapid. My tissue integrity was strong. I wasn't just up and walking in record time; I was discharged. Why? Because the work **had already** been done. When I arrived at the hospital, I was in an **optimal nutritional** state, and my body had all the necessary raw materials to sustain and rebuild itself.

Most patients show up to surgery **malnourished** in ways not every blood test captures. Their gut is compromised, their immune system is sluggish, high blood sugar is slowing down tissue repair, and they have inadequate protein intake and reserves, with healing pathways underpowered.

Mine were **overbuilt**.

How overbuilt? They could even protect me from human error, **my own errors**.

7.9   Second visit to the ER

Almost a week after my discharge, I began experiencing mild pain in the area of the operation and a low-grade fever. These were telltale signs of an **infection**. The initial stages. Off to the ER again.

A CT scan revealed an abscess, an infection near the surgical site. This was usually bad and concerning news. How could this have happened?

Showing the surgeon my two pill bottles, he quickly explained.

He had prescribed me antibiotics and pain/anti-inflammatory medication. He also explained that I was supposed to take antibiotics daily, and he specifically instructed me to use the pain medication and anti-inflammatory only when needed, as one of its side effects was an **increased risk** of abscesses forming.

I'd completely misunderstood the medication protocol. Not only that, I'd **reversed** it! I'd skipped the antibiotics and taken the anti-inflammatory daily!

Even committing this not-so-small mistake at such a critical juncture of my post-operative recovery, I only developed a **4cm** abscess, so small that it couldn't even be aspirated.

I was admitted to the hospital. I was set with IV antibiotics to sterilize the abscess. Once sterilized, the body would naturally absorb it. The total estimated stay was about five days.

Unlike my previous admission two weeks prior, I was feeling quite well, strong, and eager to return to my everyday life. So, what better way to spend my time waiting for the little abscess to disappear than to continue where I left off with the outline and start writing the story you are **reading right now**?

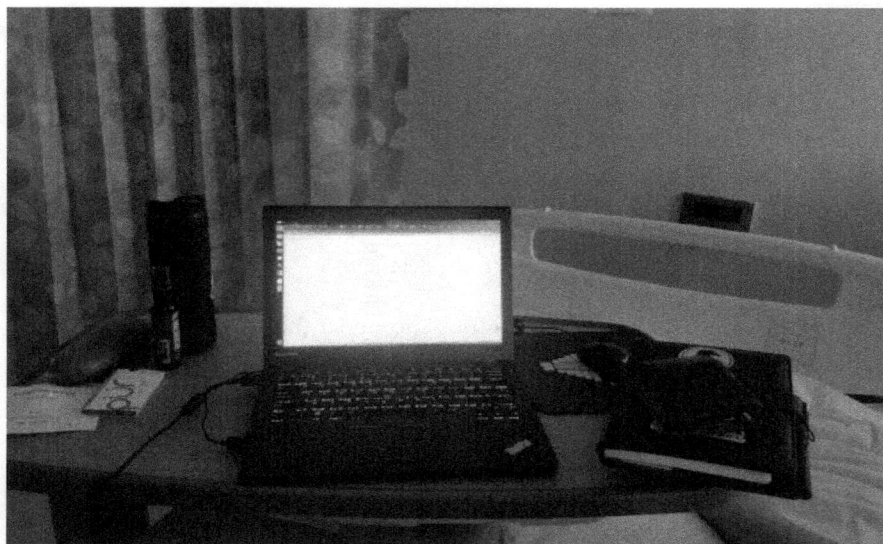

Fig. 6: Writing the first draft of the book at the hospital.

After a few days in the hospital, I was back home again in record time. That's a testament to my health protocol. It protected me, even from my own mistakes, at the **worst possible** time.

That was the result of a system I'd designed and tested for years through OpenHolter EKG recordings, symptom journals, environmental monitoring, and a customized wellness protocol that rebuilt my heart, liver, gut, hormones, inflammation response, and tissue resilience. It didn't just **optimize me**; it **saved me** more than once.

I survived because I treated my health like the most important project of my life.

I developed, tested, optimized, and shipped it to production.

8

WHY I SURVIVED

Albumin, Gut Resilience, and System Integrity

"What you think, you become. What you feel, you attract. What you imagine, you create." - Buddha

Most people believe that healing is just a matter of luck. Or youth. Or genetics.

It's not. It's systems design.

My doctors were baffled. I had just gone through a ruptured appendix, intestinal necrosis, four days of infection, and an intestinal resection that significantly altered my digestive tract. And yet, I wasn't breaking down. I wasn't suffering complications. I wasn't even struggling.

Why? Because I had **already built** the biological infrastructure to withstand catastrophe.

8.1 Stress

Let's start with stress. And not just the initial stages felt during an unknown illness but the entire spectrum of stress levels experienced from the start of the emergency to the hospital discharge.

8.1.1 Emotional

Stress is no joke. Even in normal conditions, such as working in an office, stress will affect your health. Now imagine a medical emergency scenario where your body needs every ounce of energy to heal. Still, stress is causing your body to divert energy and nutrients to areas that are not essential, such as muscles, vision, and awareness. The fight-or-flight response **prioritizes survival at the expense** of other functions, resulting in long-term effects on health.

ER patients experience high levels of stress because of the unpredictable nature of their situations, the potential for life-threatening conditions, and the often chaotic environment. Research indicates that **87%** of ER patients experience signs of high stress. This stress can lead to anxiety, fear, and even **post-traumatic stress disorder** (PTSD). [281]

Even attendants accompanying patients to the emergency department experience elevated stress levels. Research shows that up to **98%** of attendants experience stress levels that can lead to conflict, violence, and affected services. [282]

Uncertainty, lack of control, fear of bodily injury, pain, separation anxiety, inadequate communication, uncomfortable procedures, wait times, disrupted sleep and eating patterns. These would be enough to drive even a healthy individual **over the edge**.

8.1.2 Mental

Besides the physiological benefits of my changes, I've also realized the importance of nurturing a **healthier mind**. To that end, I've also explored and studied the effects of mindset, beliefs, and faith on my health. **Psychosocial** and **physiological** stress are deeply interconnected and can influence each other. This connection becomes even more critical in the context of medical rehabilitation. [283]

By embracing faith and teachings from diverse sources, including **Christianity**, [284] **Buddhism**, [285] and **Stoicism**, [286] I've cultivated a robust emotional framework that made a tangible contribution to my resilience during this medical crisis. These practices not only provided psychological support but also may have positively influenced my physiological stress responses, aiding in my recovery.

8.1.3 Metabolic

When I was admitted for emergency abdominal surgery, I was placed on a complete fast of no food or even water to be ready for surgery as soon as my Troponin levels stabilized, which took four days. What could have been a dangerous metabolic crisis became a powerful validation of the path I had taken years prior. My switch to a clean ketogenic diet rich in animal protein and fats led to metabolic conditioning.

Research shows that the heart is a **metabolically flexible** organ capable of utilizing ketones, fatty acids, and lactate, particularly during periods of stress, fasting, or injury. In the absence of glucose, the heart increases its reliance on ketone bodies, which are **more efficient** fuels that **reduce oxidative stress** and **improve mitochondrial function**. [287] This metabolic adaptation, built over time by my dietary change, made my heart more resilient and primed for the challenge of fasting and surgical trauma.

The long-term effects of my diet and eating patterns led to **mitochondrial adaptation**, resulting in increased **mitochondrial biogenesis** and **efficiency**. [288] [289] [290] In essence, my mitochondria had been trained to survive, and they did.

8.2 Albumin

Why is albumin level so important?

For starters, albumin is the most abundant circulating protein found in plasma. It is produced in the liver; therefore, it serves as a marker for **liver health**. Additionally, albumin binds and carries various substances, including **hormones**, **fatty acids**, **bilirubin**, and **drugs**, through the bloodstream.

Albumin is a major contributor to the osmotic pressure within blood vessels, primarily by preventing fluid from **leaking** out into surrounding tissues. When albumin levels are low, excess fluid leaks out of blood vessels and can cause **edema**. Low albumin levels are associated with an increased risk of **pulmonary embolism** (PE) and can also worsen the severity of PE. [291] [292] [293]

Albumin synthesis is **not** a high priority for the liver, meaning it only occurs when the body is **adequately nourished**. Inadequate nutrition, inflammation, and exposure to hepatotoxins can inhibit its production. Therefore, albumin serves as an important marker for both **nutritional status** and **inflammation**. [294]

These aspects combine to make albumin level one of the **strongest** predictors of post-surgical recovery.

Serum albumin levels have been identified as potential predictors of adverse outcomes in **abdominal surgery**, [295] more so for **intestinal resection**. [296] The decline in relative serum albumin concentration can help predict anastomotic leakage, [297] a serious and potentially life-threatening complication that may occur after surgical procedures involving intestinal reconstruction.

One paper identifies **3.4 g/dL** as the optimal threshold for predicting postoperative mortality and complications. [298]

Table 1: Optimal serum albumin cutoff (g/dL) to predict 30-day postoperative adverse events. Note: CPR - cardiopulmonary resuscitation; CVA - cerebrovascular accident; SSI - surgical site infection; DVT - deep venous thrombosis.

Outcomes	Optimal Serum Albumin Cutoff (g/dL)
Death	3.4
Cardiac Arrest Requiring CPR	3.5
Myocardial Infarction	3.7
Stroke/CVA	3.7
Reoperation	3.5
Composite Primary Adverse Events	3.5
Superficial Incisional SSI	3.7
Deep Incisional SSI	3.6
Organ/Space SSI	3.5
Wound Disruption	3.6
Pneumonia	3.4
Urinary Tract Infection	3.5
Sepsis	3.3
Septic Shock	3.4
Unplanned Intubation	3.5
On Ventilator greater than 48 Hours	3.4
Pulmonary Embolism	3.6
DVT Requiring Therapy	3.2
Acute Renal Failure	3.5
Transfusions	3.3
Unplanned Readmission	3.8
Prolonged length of stay	3.3
Composite Secondary Adverse Events	3.3

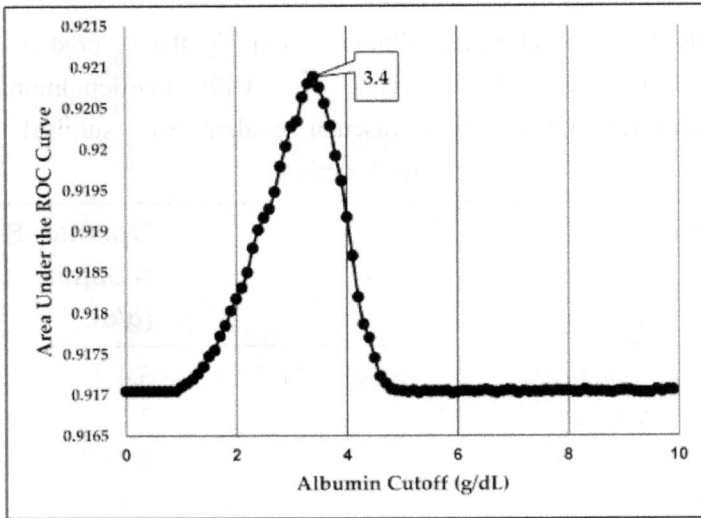

Fig. 1: Albumin cutoff (g/dL) chart.

The studies I reviewed typically report albumin levels using a threshold of **3.4 g/dL**, categorizing patients as either **hypoalbuminemic** (albumin level ≤3.4 g/dL) or **normal** (albumin level >3.4 g/dL). As a result, exact distribution data is often not provided, but it can be reasonably estimated using a normal distribution based on known means and standard deviations.

The average hospitalized patient has an albumin level ranging from **3.9** to **4.0 g/dL**. However, up to **17.6%** of patients present with **hypoalbuminemia** (≤3.4 g/dL), which is at or below the threshold commonly associated with increased risk of postoperative complications and mortality.

Mine was **5 g/dL**.

That's not just rare; it's nearly unheard of in emergency cases.

A serum albumin level of **5.0 g/dL** occurs in fewer than **1%** of cases, about **seven** patients per **1,000**.

That albumin level wasn't an accident. It was a metric I earned, day by day, plate by plate.

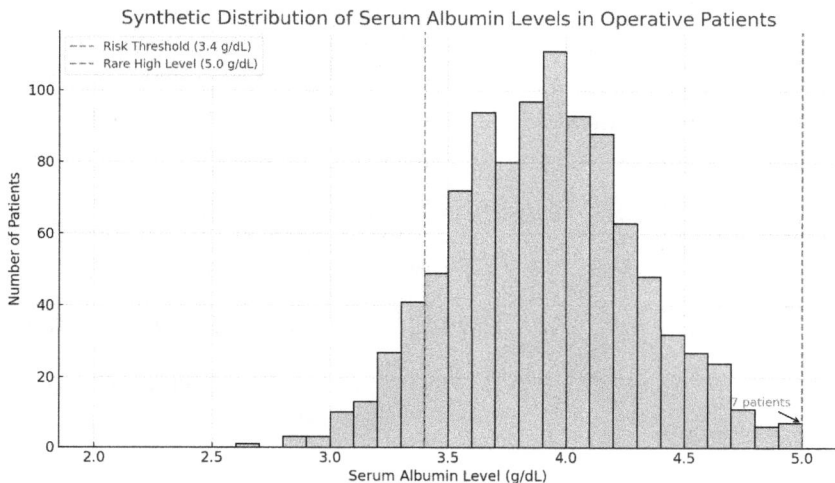

Fig. 2: A synthetic model of serum albumin distribution in operative patients, modeled with a normal distribution (mean = 3.9 g/dL, SD = 0.4).

How did I get there?

8.3 Nutrition

In the years following the development of my unique wellness protocol, I've been focusing on consuming foods with **maximum nutrient density**. I prioritized high-bioavailability proteins, such as **eggs**, **liver**, **fish**, and **red meat**. [299] I also combined a **high-protein diet** with **high-intensity** exercise, which resulted in increased albumin protein synthesis. [300]

I also avoided **inflammatory** foods that not only damaged my gut lining but also decreased albumin levels. [301] I practice **intermittent fasting** and **time-restricted eating**, which reduce systemic inflammation and improve metabolic markers.

The **low carbohydrate** aspect of my diet also reduced advanced glycation end products (AGEs). Reducing AGEs and inflammation had a protective effect on the renal endothelial cells of my kidneys, which prevented **albuminuria**. [302] Albuminuria is the presence of albumin in the urine. It's an indicator that the kidneys are not functioning correctly and that albumin, which should remain in the bloodstream, is being **leaked into the urine**.

> *You can't build resilience when you're already facing a crisis. It's a foundation you lay before adversity strikes. When the **inevitable** challenges arise, your ability to navigate them will be a **direct** reflection of the groundwork you've laid.*

I stopped believing in "common sense" and started believing in **inputs that work**.

Once I understood the importance of nutrition as a **primary factor** in achieving optimal health, everything fell into place.

8.4   Supplementation

Besides what I could obtain from food, I also started researching what I needed to add that was either missing from modern food or not bioavailable to my body due to my specific conditions or age.

All supplements improved my health in one or multiple aspects. However, here are some notable supplements. These are my recovery MVPs.

8.4.1   Zinc

Zinc supplementation over the years leading up to my surgery was a key factor in my recovery.

Before correcting the course of my health, I was suffering from Nonalcoholic steatohepatitis (NASH). NASH prevents the body from absorbing zinc effectively, leading to a zinc deficiency. Zinc deficiency, in turn, exacerbates liver inflammation, oxidative stress, and insulin resistance. [303] I saw this as a **bidirectional cycle** in which zinc deficiency contributes to the worsening of liver pathology, and liver disease disrupts zinc homeostasis.

The ketogenic diet has been shown to **reverse** hepatic steatosis and hepatic mitochondrial metabolism in nonalcoholic fatty liver disease. [304] With this diet, in conjunction with the therapeutic supplementation of zinc, I was able to **break** that vicious cycle.

Breaking that cycle allowed me to benefit from zinc's crucial role in protein metabolism and in aiding the healing process when it mattered the most.

8.4.2   Vitamin C

I take **larger amounts** of Vitamin C than recommended as an immune booster and adrenal suppressor to manage adrenal stress, reduce oxidative damage, and protect my organs and DNA. These factors have already helped me improve my heart condition.   However, Vitamin C also contributed to **many** aspects of my postoperative recovery beyond the immune boost.

Modern medicine has revolutionized the way surgeries are performed, utilizing advanced tools, improved anesthesia, and precise life-saving techniques. But to our biology, surgery is still an assault. The body doesn't know the difference between a **scalpel in a sterile operating room** and a **knife in a back alley.**

From the body's perspective, it's being cut open, fluids are lost, and tissues are disrupted. It triggers the same primal response as an injury or attack: a full-blown stress cascade involving **cortisol, catecholamines** (such as adrenaline), **inflammatory cytokines, insulin resistance,** and **hypermetabolism.**   These aren't just side effects; they're deeply wired survival responses.

This stress response is baked into the human blueprint. [305] It can't be fully turned off, not even with the best anesthesia. During this state, the body enters a catabolic state, prioritizing energy for vital organs, mobilizing blood sugar, and breaking down muscle tissue to fuel the healing process. In essence, the body goes into emergency mode to survive the insult, no matter how clean or high-tech the incision may be.

One of the most essential hormones during trauma is **cortisol**, your body's built-in stress shield. It maintains stable blood pressure, keeps inflammation in check, and provides energy when it's needed most. But surgery pushes the adrenal glands to their **limits**.

Even if your hormone levels are normal before the operation, you can still experience what's called **relative adrenal insufficiency** (RAI). [306] Relative adrenal insufficiency (RAI) means the adrenal glands are functioning, but they **can't ramp up** cortisol production enough to match the extreme stress of surgery. Without sufficient cortisol in those critical moments, recovery slows, complications increase, and things can quickly spiral out of control.

No one told me this before surgery: anesthesia doesn't just knock you out. Yes, it keeps you from feeling pain, a miracle of modern medicine. But while your mind slips into unconsciousness, your cells **don't get a free pass**.

But Vitamin C also helps here. It significantly reduces the **cellular death** caused by anesthesia. It guards vulnerable cells from the wave of oxidative stress. At higher doses, Vitamin C even blocks the very proteins that trigger apoptosis, like caspase-3. [307]

Anesthesia can have a particularly negative impact on **soft tissues**, including cartilage, tendons, and ligaments. And once cartilage is damaged, it **rarely heals well**. It has no blood supply and no reinforcement. That makes Vitamin C all the more vital because it helps build collagen, the scaffolding that cartilage depends on. [308] [309] [310] [311]

As part of changing my diet, I replaced many food additives; one of those was coffee creamer. I now use collagen powder with my morning coffee.

This change, in addition to my animal protein-based diet and consumption of bone broth, increased my net dietary intake of collagen. The higher intake of collagen, **combined** with Vitamin C, **supported** and **protected** my connective tissue during recovery from surgery. [312]

In a world where surgeries are routine, and recovery is assumed, it's easy to forget the hidden battle going on inside the body. Healing isn't a **passive process**. It's not something that "just happens". Your body needs raw materials, reinforcements, and, sometimes, a little backup.

And for me, Vitamin C was that backup, silent, powerful, and essential.

8.5   Gut health

Then there was the **gut microbiome**. Most people crash on antibiotics. Their digestion shuts down. They experience bloating, constipation, anxiety, or mental fog. But my gut didn't skip a beat.

Why?

Because I hadn't just fed myself, I'd fed my microbes.

My gut was so healthy that unbeknownst to me, I had been living with **chronic appendicopathy** for years. [313] Still, I led a normal life with just rare, occasional faint Right Lower Quadrant (RLQ) pain and no IBS. My appendix was compromised, and my diet had delayed the appendicitis by years. [314] [315]

Maintaining a healthy intestinal flora even had positive effects on my **neurological** and **mental** health. There is a bidirectional relationship between the gut microbiome and brain functionality. [316] A healthier and calmer mind will enhance outcomes during uncertain times. Decision-making, emotional regulation, and resilience are all improved.

In the worst case, my diet extended my life considerably and improved its quality.

But I experienced the **best-case** scenario; my diet saved my life.

Since reformulating my diet, I have avoided processed foods and synthetic sweeteners. I included small amounts of fermented foods, such as sauerkraut, kimchi, kombucha, and real yogurt, as well as kefir. By consistently nourishing it and avoiding sugar spikes and gut-permeating seed oils, I developed a robust and adaptable microbiome, which brought clarity and consistency to my gut health. In nature, **you are either a bacteria** or a **host for bacteria**. I became the best host for the best kind of bacteria. This protected me from **antibiotic-resistant** bacteria and antibiotic-resistant **horizontal gene transfer** from within my own body.

When the antibiotics arrived, I had the resilience to bounce back quickly.

8.6 Pain

Even my **pain tolerance** shocked the staff and my caretakers.

I was authorized IV morphine every four hours. Instead, I managed the pain with minimal medication. Once the pain did not increase my blood pressure, I stopped all painkillers. The discomfort was real, but it was manageable. Years of self-regulation, martial arts, fasting, cold exposure, and high-symptom tolerance, achieved through gut repair, gave me the mindset and neurological tools to handle stress without panic.

Plus, I had an ally. Another unexpected benefit of Vitamin C is its role in **pain modulation**.

Vitamin C is an **Antinociception**, meaning it reduces pain or the blocking of the detection of a painful stimulus by sensory neurons. [317] My discipline, along with this benefit, explains my significant postoperative reduced pain severity and low dependency on opioid analgesics.

Mentally, my relationship with pain had also changed long ago. But thanks to a book by Norman Cousins and his own experience battling a deadly medical condition, [318] I took this to a new level. I no longer saw pain as a punishing sensation but as a necessary feedback system. One that is not just good but **essential** for healing.

8.7   Bottom line

They kept asking, "*Why is your body recovering so fast?*" Because I treated my body like a system under active development. I stress-tested, optimized, and invested in it the way I would in a product going into production.

You can't build resilience when you're already facing a crisis. It's a foundation you lay before adversity strikes. When the **inevitable** challenges arise, your ability to navigate them will be a **direct** reflection of the groundwork you've laid.

I was not strong out of nowhere. I prepared for the future problems **yesterday**, and they had arrived. Just as I would when developing and improving a system, I profiled my health. I focused on what determines the quality of the system: the integrity indicators.

Instead of pursuing big muscles and staring at myself in the mirror, I concentrated on developing stamina, flexibility, a focused mind, clear skin, a steady heart rate, a calm gut, and a flat stomach. These are the **fundamental indicators** of your **internal integrity**, your **longevity markers**.

I didn't survive that surgery by accident.

I survived it because I had already **developed, applied, tested,** and **shipped** all the **patches to fix my health**.

9

THE FUTURE OF DIY HEALTH

Lessons for Developers and Makers

"As each has received a gift, use it to serve one another." - 1 Peter 4:10

You don't need a medical degree to understand your body; you simply need to be a **systems thinker**.

After navigating a journey marked by heart issues, gut dysfunction, emergency surgery, and full recovery, I've come to one resounding conclusion: health is not a mystery; **it's a system**. And like any system, it can observed, tested, logged, and debugged.

As a developer, I'd been accustomed to dealing with complex systems daily. When software broke, I didn't panic; instead, I gathered logs, identified root causes, traced variables, and iterated until the issue was resolved.

I didn't rely on wishful thinking or prayer for uptime and reliability; I engineered it.

So why do we treat our bodies so differently?

We trust **food labels**, **government guidelines**, **social media influencers**, and **marketing hype**. We trust these sources **more** than we trust our internal metrics. We outsource our well-being to others who may not fully comprehend our health in the context of our daily lives.

That's not a **judgment**. It's a statement of fact, the unfortunate default.

But it doesn't have to be.

You don't need a **crisis** to justify taking control of **your health**. You don't require a diagnosis, nor do you need access to cutting-edge tools. All you need is a brain trained to solve problems and a body that's waiting to be understood.

The future of health **won't** emerge from institutions bound by regulations and the paradigms set by insurance companies; instead, it will come from individuals, engineers, tinkerers, skeptics, and makers who take **ownership** of their well-being with an open mind and a willingness to learn.

You don't need **permission** to embark on this journey. The only thing you need is a process, one that involves treating your body as the most critical project you'll ever maintain. Once you stop viewing your health as a **mystery**, everything changes.

Just like it did for me.

As it did also for my oldest son.

Then for my wife, and finally for our youngest son.

And as it has done for others, as I later learned.

After my family's health recovery, that was the most **surprising** and **rewarding** outcome of building the OpenHolter and embarking on this wellness journey. Realizing it didn't just help me, but also others.

It's been incredible to see so many projects **replicate** and **expand** on the

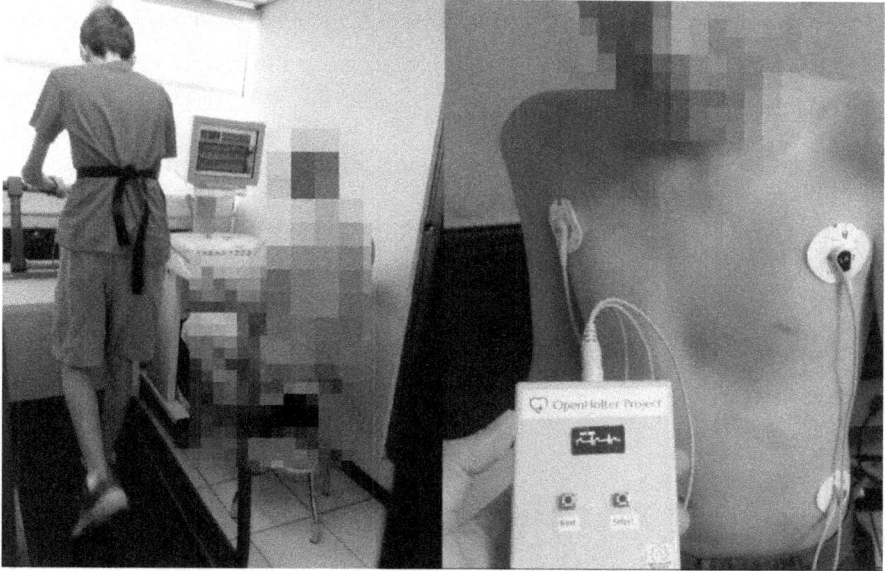

Fig. 1: My oldest son started experiencing symptoms similar to mine. The OpenHolter also became a part of this diagnosis and recovery.

OpenHolter, adding features like **Bluetooth**, **mobile apps**, and even early **AI models for signal interpretation**. [319]

What began as a means to monitor my heart health sparked a small revolution, a new mindset that emphasizes **patient empowerment** and **self-directed recovery**.

This shift in perspective extends far beyond DIY heart monitoring; it's about recognizing that healthcare is not solely the domain of professionals but rather a **shared responsibility** between patients and caregivers.

Yes, patients have the **responsibility** of being **active participants** in their recovery.

The journey of wellness is not a return to a state of unattainable, **100% perfect** health; that is not the point. It is rather a continuous process of discovery, growth, and iterative improvement.

If you've read this far, you already know what you need to do: reclaim control over your health. Regardless of your situation or condition, **you can do it** just as I did.

And just like me, all you need is **motivation** and **information**.

Do it without relying on guesswork or quick fixes. But with data, intention, and the same mindset you bring to your most critical projects:

- **Build Observability.** Track the metrics that matter most: food intake, symptoms, sleep patterns, heart rate, energy levels, and mood. Log enough data to identify connections between seemingly unrelated factors.

- **Instrument Your System.** Utilize tools like the OpenHolter, wearables, or even manual logs to capture the raw signals your body sends. These signals are there; you just need a means to listen to them.

- **Create Your Feedback Loop.** Integrate your inputs with your outputs. What happens when you consume a specific food? How does it affect your sleep patterns? What impact does stress have on your digestive system? Make this connection accessible and actionable.

- **Run Safe Experiments.** Change one variable at a time, observe the effects, and roll back if necessary. Trust the trends, not the fads; focus on making incremental progress rather than seeking instant gratification.

- **Refactor Ruthlessly.** When something isn't working, cut it without justification or defense. Your health doesn't care about your beliefs or biases; only your inputs have the power to shape your well-being.

- **Engineer Resilience.** Stop chasing "perfect" and focus on building systems that can recover from setbacks rather than merely improving performance under ideal conditions.

And most importantly:

Start now.

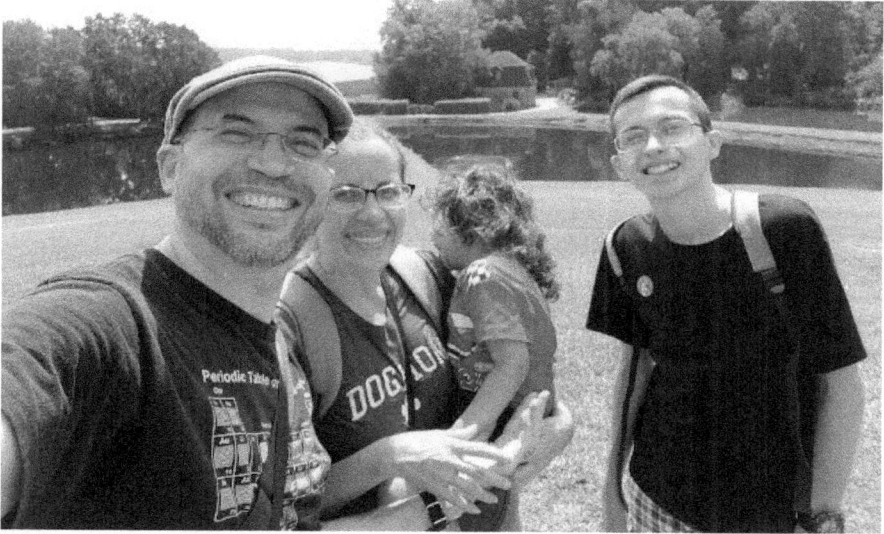

Fig. 2: Regain your health, mobility, and independence for you and yours.

ABOUT THE AUTHOR

Roberto Rosario is a technologist, martial artist, and software developer with over three decades of professional experience, as well as a health innovator who has turned personal adversity into a blueprint for self-healing.

His journey in computing began in the early 1980s when he first delved into the world of computers on platforms like the TRS-80 and Commodore 64. As an early adopter of Linux in the 1990s, he fell in love with the free and open-source mindset. Understanding its potential, he founded several groups and quickly became a prominent advocate for free and open-source software and its philosophy.

Years later, as Director of Software Development for the Government of Puerto Rico, he would do the same for the government of the island by spearheading initiatives that harnessed the power of free and open-source software as a public policy, driving transparency through official portals, government technology events, and IT internship programs.

Through the years, Rosario has also lent his support to several notable Django and Python projects and communities, both financially and organizationally.

As a speaker and ambassador, he has appeared at numerous international conferences and media outlets, promoting the importance of open data, digital rights, and the social value of technology.

Throughout his career, Rosario has conceived and contributed to numerous software projects, many of which have garnered global recognition as open-source initiatives. His work spans diverse sectors, including document management, education, medical technology, embedded systems, geospatial technologies, statistics, privacy and free speech, business intelligence, analytics, open legislation, and even the preservation and emulation of vintage hardware.

He is best known for creating Mayan EDMS, a widely adopted open-source electronic document management system used by governments, universities, and enterprises worldwide. Rosario has also authored "Exploring Mayan EDMS: The Definitive Guide", showcasing his expertise in the field of electronic document management.

He now shares his journey to inspire others to take control of their health through an engineer's mindset.

BIBLIOGRAPHY

[1]   Christopher Amann, Andrea Austin, and Sherri Rudinsky. Valentino's syndrome: a life-threatening mimic of acute appendicitis. *Clinical Practice and Cases in Emergency Medicine*, 1(1):44–46, February 2017. URL: http://dx.doi.org/10.5811/cpcem.2016.11.32571, doi:10.5811/cpcem.2016.11.32571.

[2]   Robert A. Kyle, David P. Steensma, and Marc A. Shampo. Barry James Marshall—discovery of helicobacter pylori as a cause of peptic ulcer. *Mayo Clinic Proceedings*, May 2016. doi:10.1016/j.mayocp.2016.01.025.

[3]   Robert A. Schwartz, Christopher A. Janusz, and Camila K. Janniger. Seborrheic dermatitis: An overview. Jul 2006. URL: https://www.aafp.org/pubs/afp/issues/2006/0701/p125.html.

[4]   Elocon Cream - Patient Information Leaflet (PIL) - (emc) | 78. URL: https://www.medicines.org.uk/emc/product/78/pil.

[5]   Belinda Sheary. Steroid Withdrawal Effects Following Long-term Topical Corticosteroid Use. *Dermatitis*, 29(4):213–218, July 2018. URL: http://dx.doi.org/10.1097/DER.0000000000000387, doi:10.1097/der.0000000000000387.

[6]   Jayasree BASIVIREDDY, Molly JACOB, and Kunissery A. BALASUBRAMANIAN. Oral glutamine attenuates indomethacin-induced small intestinal damage. *Clinical Science*, 107(3):281–289, August 2004. URL: http://dx.doi.org/10.1042/CS20030390, doi:10.1042/cs20030390.

[7]   E. DEN HOND, PEETERS, HIELE, BULTEEL, GHOOS, and RUTGEERTS. Effect of glutamine on the intestinal permeability changes induced by indomethacin in humans. *Alimentary Pharmacology & Therapeutics*, 13(5):679–685, May 1999. URL: http://dx.doi.org/10.1046/j.1365-2036.1999.00523.x, doi:10.1046/j.1365-2036.1999.00523.x.

[8]   Abigail Davis and John Robson. The dangers of NSAIDs: look both ways. *British Journal of General Practice*, 66(645):172–173, March 2016. URL: http://dx.doi.org/10.3399/bjgp16X684433, doi:10.3399/bjgp16x684433.

[9]   Department of Clinical Pharmacology. Analgesics and glutathione : American Journal of Therapeutics. URL: https://journals.lww.com/americantherapeutics/Abstract/2002/05000/Analgesics_and_Glutathione.8.aspx.

[10]   Gastroesophageal reflux disease (GERD). Apr 2025. URL: https://www.mayoclinic.org/diseases-conditions/gerd/symptoms-causes/syc-20361940.

[11]   Douglas C. Wolf. Dysphagia. Jan 1990. URL: https://www.ncbi.nlm.nih.gov/books/NBK408/.

[12]   Andrew C Dukowicz, Brian E Lacy, and Gary M Levine. Small intestinal bacterial overgrowth: a comprehensive review. *Gastroenterology & hepatology*, 3(2):112, 2007.

[13]   Paulina Roszkowska, Emilia Klimczak, Ewa Ostrycharz, Aleksandra Rączka, Iwona Wojciechowska-Koszko, Andrzej Dybus, Yeong-

Hsiang Cheng, Yu-Hsiang Yu, Szymon Mazgaj, and Beata Hukowska-Szematowicz. Small Intestinal Bacterial Overgrowth (SIBO) and Twelve Groups of Related Diseases—Current State of Knowledge. *Biomedicines*, 2024. URL: https://www.mdpi.com/2227-9059/12/5/1030, doi:10.3390/biomedicines12051030.

[14] Anna Gudan, Dominika Jamioł-Milc, Victoria Hawryłkowicz, Karolina Skonieczna-Żydecka, and Ewa Stachowska. The Prevalence of Small Intestinal Bacterial Overgrowth in Patients with Non-Alcoholic Liver Diseases: NAFLD, NASH, Fibrosis, Cirrhosis—A Systematic Review, Meta-Analysis and Meta-Regression. *Nutrients*, 2022. URL: https://www.mdpi.com/2072-6643/14/24/5261, doi:10.3390/nu14245261.

[15] Arun J. Sanyal. AGA technical review on nonalcoholic fatty liver disease. *Gastroenterology*, 123(5):1705–1725, November 2002. URL: http://dx.doi.org/10.1053/gast.2002.36572, doi:10.1053/gast.2002.36572.

[16] Arjun Kalra, Ekrem Yetiskul, Chase J. Wehrle, and Faiz Tuma. *Physiology, Liver*. StatPearls Publishing, Treasure Island (FL), 2025. URL: http://europepmc.org/books/NBK535438.

[17] Evangelia Makri, Antonis Goulas, and Stergios A. Polyzos. Epidemiology, Pathogenesis, Diagnosis and Emerging Treatment of Nonalcoholic Fatty Liver Disease. *Archives of Medical Research*, 52(1):25–37, 2021. URL: https://www.sciencedirect.com/science/article/pii/S0188440920322396, doi:https://doi.org/10.1016/j.arcmed.2020.11.010.

[18] K Gilani and Mohtaram Vafakhah. Hypoxia: a review. *Journal of Paramedical Sciences (JPS)*, 2010. URL: https://www.sid.ir/EN/VEWSSID/J_pdf/127220100209.pdf.

[19] Atrial fibrillation ablation. Apr 2024. URL: https://www.mayoclinic.org/tests-procedures/atrial-fibrillation-ablation/about/pac-20384969.

[20] Cleveland Clinic medical professional. How does cardiac ablation work? Dec 2024. URL: https://my.clevelandclinic.org/health/trea tments/16851-catheter-ablation.

[21] "The OpenHolter project: DIY Cardiometry with Arduino and Django." by Roberto Rosario. URL: https://www.youtube.com/wa tch?v=rubzEAojf-k.

[22] Roberto Rosario. OpenHolter project: D.I.Y. electrocardiography using Arduino and Django. URL: https://speakerdeck.com/silora ptor/openholter-project-d-dot-i-y-electrocardiography-using-ardui no-and-django.

[23] Arduino Nano SKU A000005. URL: https://docs.arduino.cc/resource s/datasheets/A000005-datasheet.pdf.

[24] ATMEGA328P datasheet. URL: https://ww1.microchip.com/downlo ads/en/DeviceDoc/Atmel-7810-Automotive-Microcontrollers-ATm ega328P_Datasheet.pdf.

[25] Piyu Dhaker. Introduction to SPI interface. URL: https://www.analog .com/en/resources/analog-dialogue/articles/introduction-to-spi-inter face.html.

[26] Joseph Wu. Application Note A Basic Guide to I2C. URL: https://ww w.ti.com/lit/an/sbaa565/sbaa565.pdf.

[27] Agus Kurniawan. *IoT Projects with Arduino Nano 33 BLE Sense.* Apress, 2021. URL: http://dx.doi.org/10.1007/978-1-4842-6458-4, doi:10.1007/978-1-4842-6458-4.

[28] J. Lee, M.S. Lee, M. Jang, and J.-M. Lim. Comparison of Arduino Nano and Due processors for time-based data acquisition for low-cost mobile radiation detection system. *Journal of Instrumentation*, 17(03):P03015, March 2022. URL: http://dx.doi.org/10.1088/174 8-0221/17/03/P03015, doi:10.1088/1748-0221/17/03/p03015.

[29] AD8232 Single-Lead, Heart Rate Monitor Front End Data Sheet. URL: https://www.analog.com/media/en/technical-documentation/data-sheets/ad8232.pdf.

[30] DS3231 Extremely Accurate I2C-Integrated RTC/TCXO/Crystal. URL: https://www.analog.com/media/en/technical-documentation/data-sheets/ds3231.pdf.

[31] Solomon Systech Limited Advance Information SSD1306 128 x 64 Dot Matrix OLED/PLED Segment/Common Driver with Controller. URL: https://soldered.com/productdata/2022/03/Soldered_SSD1306_datasheet.pdf.

[32] Olikraus. Olikraus/U8g2_Arduino: U8glib V2 Library for Arduino. URL: https://github.com/olikraus/U8g2_Arduino.

[33] ANSI/AAMI EC53:2013 (R2020) - ECG trunk cables and patient leadwires. URL: https://webstore.ansi.org/standards/aami/ansiaamiec532013r2020.

[34] Brian Young. New standards for ECG equipment. *Journal of Electrocardiology*, 57:S1–S4, November 2019. URL: http://dx.doi.org/10.1016/j.jelectrocard.2019.07.013, doi:10.1016/j.jelectrocard.2019.07.013.

[35] Understanding Lithium-Ion Technology.

[36] Bill Greiman. Greiman/SDFAT: Arduino FAT16/FAT32 Exfat Library. URL: https://github.com/greiman/SdFat.

[37] John G Bradley and Kathy A Davis. Orthostatic hypotension. *American family physician*, 68(12):2393–2399, 2003.

[38] Julian M. Stewart, Shahid Javaid, Tyler Fialkoff, Brianna Tuma-Marcella, Paul Visintainer, Courtney Terilli, and Marvin S. Medow. Initial Orthostatic Hypotension Causes (Transient) Postural Tachycardia. *JACC*, 74(9):1271–1273, 2019. URL: https://www.jacc.org/doi/abs/10.1016/j.jacc.2019.06.054,

arXiv:https://www.jacc.org/doi/pdf/10.1016/j.jacc.2019.06.054, doi:10.1016/j.jacc.2019.06.054.

[39] Laura Coudrey. The Troponins. *Archives of Internal Medicine*, 158(11):1173, June 1998. URL: http://dx.doi.org/10.1001/archint e.158.11.1173, doi:10.1001/archinte.158.11.1173.

[40] Vinay S. Mahajan and Petr Jarolim. How to Interpret Elevated Cardiac Troponin Levels. *Circulation*, 124(21):2350–2354, November 2011. URL: http://dx.doi.org/10.1161/CIRCULATIONAHA.111.023697, doi:10.1161/circulationaha.111.023697.

[41] Allen Jeremias and C. Michael Gibson. Narrative Review: Alternative Causes for Elevated Cardiac Troponin Levels when Acute Coronary Syndromes Are Excluded. *Annals of Internal Medicine*, 142(9):786–791, May 2005. URL: http://dx.doi.org/10.7326/0003-4819-142-9-2 00505030-00015, doi:10.7326/0003-4819-142-9-200505030-00015.

[42] Farman Ali, Khurram Arshad, Susan Szpunar, and Edouard Daher. Elevated Troponins and Diagnosis of Non-ST-Elevation Myocardial Infarction in the Emergency Department. *Cureus*, May 2024. URL: http://dx.doi.org/10.7759/cureus.59910, doi:10.7759/cureus.59910.

[43] Grigorios Avdikos, George Michas, and Stephen W. Smith. From Q/Non-Q Myocardial Infarction to STEMI/NSTEMI: Why It's Time to Consider Another Simplified Dichotomy; a Narrative Literature Review. *Archives of Academic Emergency Medicine*, 10(1):e78, October 2022. URL: https://doi.org/10.22037/aaem.v10i1.1783, doi:10.22037/aaem.v10i1.1783.

[44] D. Rott and D. Leibowitz. STEMI and NSTEMI are two distinct pathophysiological entities. *European Heart Journal*, 28(21):2685–2685, October 2007. URL: http://dx.doi.org/10.1093/eurheartj/e hm368, doi:10.1093/eurheartj/ehm368.

[45]   A. W. J. van 't Hof and E. Badings. NSTEMI treatment: should we always follow the guidelines? *Netherlands Heart Journal*, 27(4):171–175, March 2019. URL: http://dx.doi.org/10.1007/s12471-019-124 4-3, doi:10.1007/s12471-019-1244-3.

[46]   Stefano Govoni, Alessia Pascale, Marialaura Amadio, Laura Calvillo, Emilia D'Elia, Cristina Cereda, Piercarlo Fantucci, Mauro Ceroni, and Emilio Vanoli. NGF and heart: Is there a role in heart disease? *Pharmacological Research*, 63(4):266–277, 2011. URL: https://ww w.sciencedirect.com/science/article/pii/S1043661810002549, doi:https://doi.org/10.1016/j.phrs.2010.12.017.

[47]   R. ROSARIO. *Exploring Mayan EDMS: The Definitive Guide for Mayan EDMS Version 3.2.* Amazon Digital Services LLC - Kdp, 2019. ISBN 9798316928941. URL: https://books.google.com.pr/books?id =hmBY0QEACAAJ.

[48]   Roberto Rosario. Mayan EDMS.

[49]   Cookiecutter. Cookiecutter/Cookiecutter-Django: Cookiecutter Django is a framework for jumpstarting production-ready django projects quickly. URL: https://github.com/cookiecutter/cookiecutter -django.

[50]   Mayan EDMS Cookiecutter: A cookiecutter template for creating Mayan EDMS apps quickly. URL: https://gitlab.com/mayan-edm s/cookiecutter-mayan.

[51]   Features - Mayan EDMS 4.9.1 documentation. Jan 2025. URL: https: //docs.mayan-edms.com/parts/features.html.

[52]   Hurricane Maria Leaves Puerto Rico Facing Months Without Power, url=https://www.nbcnews.com/news/weather/hurricane-maria-leaves-puerto-rico-facing-months-without-power-n803326, journal=NBCNews.com, publisher=NBCUniversal News Group, year=2017, month=Sep.

[53] FEMA Mismanaged the Commodity Distribution Process in Response to Hurricanes Irma and Maria. Sep 2020. URL: https://www.oig.dhs.gov/sites/default/files/assets/2020-09/OIG-20-76-Sep20.pdf.

[54] Suicide rates spike in Puerto Rico, five months after Maria, url=https://www.nbcnews.com/storyline/puerto-rico-crisis/suicide-rates-spike-puerto-rico-five-months-after-maria-n849666, journal=NBCNews.com, publisher=NBCUniversal News Group, year=2018, month=Feb.

[55] Death toll in Puerto Rico from Hurricane Maria officially raised to 2,975 from 64, url=https://abcnews.go.com/US/death-toll-hurricane-maria-3000-puerto-rico-study/story?id=57179291, journal=ABC News, publisher=ABC News Network.

[56] Nishant Kishore, Domingo Marqués, Ayesha Mahmud, Mathew V. Kiang, Irmary Rodriguez, Arlan Fuller, Peggy Ebner, Cecilia Sorensen, Fabio Racy, Jay Lemery, Leslie Maas, Jennifer Leaning, Rafael A. Irizarry, Satchit Balsari, and Caroline O. Buckee. Mortality in Puerto Rico after Hurricane Maria. *New England Journal of Medicine*, 379(2):162–170, July 2018. URL: http://dx.doi.org/10.1056/NEJMsa1803972, doi:10.1056/nejmsa1803972.

[57] Food Justice in Puerto Rico. Dec 2022. URL: https://puertoricoreport.com/food-justice-in-puerto-rico/.

[58] Peter Marsters and Trevor Houser. America's Biggest Blackout. Oct 2017. URL: https://rhg.com/research/americas-biggest-blackout-2/.

[59] Roberto Rosario. Solar powered microservers for a post-hurricane Maria Puerto Rico. May 2018. URL: https://medium.com/@siloraptor/solar-powered-microservers-for-a-post-hurricane-maria-puerto-rico-ca83027d20ac.

[60] Roberto Rosario. Adding a remote serial console to an odroid C2. Jun 2018. URL: https://medium.com/@siloraptor/adding-a-remote-seria

l-console-to-an-odroid-c2-87f002ab6ba0.

[61]   Yuhui Deng. Deconstructing Network Attached Storage systems. *Journal of Network and Computer Applications*, 32(5):1064–1072, September 2009. URL: http://dx.doi.org/10.1016/j.jnca.2009.02.006, doi:10.1016/j.jnca.2009.02.006.

[62]   GlusterFS Documentation. URL: https://docs.gluster.org/en/latest/.

[63]   Roberto Rosario. Self hosted enterprise document server using Mayan EDMS 3.0 and an odroid HC1. Jul 2018. URL: https://medium.com /@siloraptor/building-and-installing-mayan-edms-3-0-release-candi date-on-the-odroid-hc1-18aafdeb2f17.

[64]   Endel Tulving and Neal Kroll. Novelty assessment in the brain and long-term memory encoding. *Psychonomic Bulletin & Review*, 2(3):387–390, September 1995. URL: http://dx.doi.org/10.3758/BF0 3210977, doi:10.3758/bf03210977.

[65]   Cláuvin Almeida, Marcos Kalinowski, Anderson Uchôa, and Bruno Feijó. Negative effects of gamification in education software: Systematic mapping and practitioner perceptions. *Information and Software Technology*, 156:107142, April 2023. URL: http://dx.doi.o rg/10.1016/j.infsof.2022.107142, doi:10.1016/j.infsof.2022.107142.

[66]   Lasse Hakulinen, Tapio Auvinen, and Ari Korhonen. The Effect of Achievement Badges on Students' Behavior: An Empirical Study in a University-Level Computer Science Course. *International Journal of Emerging Technologies in Learning (iJET)*, 10(1):pp. 18–29, Feb. 2015. URL: https://online-journals.org/index.php/i-jet/article/view/ 4221, doi:10.3991/ijet.v10i1.4221.

[67]   Roberto Rosario. An educational retro game using only python? challenge accepted! URL: https://speakerdeck.com/siloraptor/a n-educational-retro-game-using-only-python-challenge-accepted.

[68] Yuji Matsuzawa, Iichiro Shimomura, Tadashi Nakamura, Yoshiaki Keno, Kasuaki Kotani, and Katsuto Tokunaga. Pathophysiology and Pathogenesis of Visceral Fat Obesity. *Obesity Research*, September 1995. URL: http://dx.doi.org/10.1002/j.1550-8528.1995.tb00462.x, doi:10.1002/j.1550-8528.1995.tb00462.x.

[69] David van der Poorten, Kerry-Lee Milner, Jason Hui, Alexander Hodge, Michael I. Trenell, James G. Kench, Roslyn London, Tony Peduto, Donald J. Chisholm, and Jacob George. Visceral Fat: A Key Mediator of Steatohepatitis in Metabolic Liver Disease. *Hepatology*, 48(2):449–457, August 2008. URL: http://dx.doi.org/10.1002/hep.22350, doi:10.1002/hep.22350.

[70] Jennifer L. Kuk, Peter T. Katzmarzyk, Milton Z. Nichaman, Timothy S. Church, Steven N. Blair, and Robert Ross. Visceral Fat Is an Independent Predictor of All-cause Mortality in Men. *Obesity*, 14(2):336–341, February 2006. URL: http://dx.doi.org/10.1038/oby.2006.43, doi:10.1038/oby.2006.43.

[71] Ingrid Lofgren, Kristin Herron, Tosca Zern, Kristy West, Madhu Patalay, Sung I. Koo, Maria Luz Fernandez, and Neil S. Shachter. Waist Circumference Is a Better Predictor than Body Mass Index of Coronary Heart Disease Risk in Overweight Premenopausal Women. *The Journal of Nutrition*, 134(5):1071–1076, May 2004. URL: http://dx.doi.org/10.1093/jn/134.5.1071, doi:10.1093/jn/134.5.1071.

[72] Jindong Wu, Jiantao Weng, Bing Xia, Yujie Zhao, and Qiuji Song. The Synergistic Effect of PM2.5 and CO_2 Concentrations on Occupant Satisfaction and Work Productivity in a Meeting Room. *International Journal of Environmental Research and Public Health*, 18(8):4109, April 2021. URL: http://dx.doi.org/10.3390/ijerph18084109, doi:10.3390/ijerph18084109.

[73] Dan Norbäck and Klas Nordström. Sick building syndrome in relation to air exchange rate, CO_2, room temperature and relative air

humidity in university computer classrooms: an experimental study. *International Archives of Occupational and Environmental Health*, 82(1):21–30, February 2008. URL: http://dx.doi.org/10.1007/s00 420-008-0301-9, doi:10.1007/s00420-008-0301-9.

[74] Carbon Dioxide Health Hazard Information Sheet. URL: https://ww w.fsis.usda.gov/sites/default/files/media_file/2020-08/Carbon-Dioxi de.pdf.

[75] Rui Wang, Wei Li, Jianfeng Gao, Chaoyi Zhao, Jiazheng Zhang, Qingfeng Bie, Mingjie Zhang, and Xinchang Chen. The Influence of Bedroom CO2 Concentration on Sleep Quality. *Buildings*, 13(11):2768, November 2023. URL: http://dx.doi.org/10.3390/bui ldings13112768, doi:10.3390/buildings13112768.

[76] HENRY D. COVELLI, J. WAYLON BLACK, MICHAEL S. OLSEN, and JEROME F. BEEKMAN. Respiratory Failure Precipitated by High Carbohydrate Loads. *Annals of Internal Medicine*, 95(5):579–581, November 1981. URL: http://dx.doi.org/10.7326/0003-4819-9 5-5-579, doi:10.7326/0003-4819-95-5-579.

[77] Bo Lönnerdal. Phytic acid–trace element (Zn, Cu, Mn) interactions. *International Journal of Food Science and Technology*, 37(7):749–758, September 2002. URL: http://dx.doi.org/10.1046/j.1365-262 1.2002.00640.x, doi:10.1046/j.1365-2621.2002.00640.x.

[78] Luisa Bertin, Miriana Zanconato, Martina Crepaldi, Giovanni Marasco, Cesare Cremon, Giovanni Barbara, Brigida Barberio, Fabiana Zingone, and Edoardo Vincenzo Savarino. The Role of the FODMAP Diet in IBS. *Nutrients*, 16(3):370, January 2024. URL: http://dx.doi.org/10.3390/nu16030370, doi:10.3390/nu16030370.

[79] Tao Gong, Xiaqiong Wang, Yanqing Yang, Yiqing Yan, Chenggong Yu, Rongbin Zhou, and Wei Jiang. Plant Lectins Activate the NLRP3 Inflammasome To Promote Inflammatory Disorders. *The Journal of*

Immunology, 198(5):2082–2092, March 2017. URL: http://dx.doi.org /10.4049/jimmunol.1600145, doi:10.4049/jimmunol.1600145.

[80] Ilka M Vasconcelos and José Tadeu A Oliveira. Antinutritional properties of plant lectins. *Toxicon*, 44(4):385–403, September 2004. URL: http://dx.doi.org/10.1016/j.toxicon.2004.05.005, doi:10.1016/j.toxicon.2004.05.005.

[81] K.E. Akande, U.D. Doma, H.O. Agu, and H.M. Adamu. Major Antinutrients Found in Plant Protein Sources: Their Effect on Nutrition. *Pakistan Journal of Nutrition*, 9(8):827–832, July 2010. URL: http://dx.doi.org/10.3923/pjn.2010.827.832, doi:10.3923/pjn.2010.827.832.

[82] J.H. Kellogg. *Plain Facts for Old and Young*. Segner & Condit, 1881. URL: https://books.google.com.pr/books?id=c3EXAQAAMAAJ.

[83] Oct 1906. URL: https://news.google.com/newspapers?nid=J-ba04z tB30C&dat=19061019&printsec=frontpage.

[84] Oct 1906. URL: https://www.newspapers.com/image/356466758.

[85] Jan 1907. URL: https://www.newspapers.com/image/168433688.

[86] THOMAS GREEN. Tricksters and the Marketing of Breakfast Cereals. *The Journal of Popular Culture*, 40(1):49–68, January 2007. URL: http://dx.doi.org/10.1111/j.1540-5931.2007.00353.x, doi:10.1111/j.1540-5931.2007.00353.x.

[87] Deborah M. Thomson. Marshmallow Power and Frooty Treasures: Disciplining the Child Consumer through Online Cereal Advergaming. *Critical Studies in Media Communication*, 27(5):438–454, December 2010. URL: http://dx.doi.org/10.1080/15295030903583648, doi:10.1080/15295030903583648.

[88] Lin Bian and Ellen M. Markman. Why do we eat cereal but not lamb chops at breakfast? Investigating Americans' beliefs about breakfast

foods. *Appetite*, 144:104458, January 2020. URL: http://dx.doi.org/1
0.1016/j.appet.2019.104458, doi:10.1016/j.appet.2019.104458.

[89]   C.E. Blake, C.A. Bisogni, J. Sobal, C.M. Devine, and M. Jastran.
Classifying foods in contexts: How adults categorize foods for
different eating settings. *Appetite*, 49(2):500–510, September 2007.
URL: http://dx.doi.org/10.1016/j.appet.2007.03.009,
doi:10.1016/j.appet.2007.03.009.

[90]   Devina Wadhera and Elizabeth D. Capaldi. Categorization of foods
as "snack" and "meal" by college students. *Appetite*, 58(3):882–888,
June 2012. URL: http://dx.doi.org/10.1016/j.appet.2012.02.006,
doi:10.1016/j.appet.2012.02.006.

[91]   Ikuko Kamada, Laurence Truman, Justine Bold, and Denise
Mortimore. The impact of breakfast in metabolic and digestive health.
Gastroenterology and hepatology from bed to bench, 4(2):76, 2011.
URL: https://pmc.ncbi.nlm.nih.gov/articles/PMC4017414/.

[92]   Lin Bian and Ellen M. Markman. What should we eat for breakfast?
American and Chinese children's prescriptive judgments about
breakfast foods. *Cognitive Development*, 54:100873, April 2020.
URL: http://dx.doi.org/10.1016/j.cogdev.2020.100873,
doi:10.1016/j.cogdev.2020.100873.

[93]   Maira Bes-Rastrollo, Matthias B. Schulze, Miguel Ruiz-Canela, and
Miguel A. Martinez-Gonzalez. Financial Conflicts of Interest and
Reporting Bias Regarding the Association between Sugar-Sweetened
Beverages and Weight Gain: A Systematic Review of Systematic
Reviews. *PLoS Medicine*, 10(12):e1001578, December 2013. URL:
http://dx.doi.org/10.1371/journal.pmed.1001578,
doi:10.1371/journal.pmed.1001578.

[94]   Dean Schillinger, Jessica Tran, Christina Mangurian, and Cristin
Kearns. Do Sugar-Sweetened Beverages Cause Obesity and Diabetes?
Industry and the Manufacture of Scientific Controversy. *Annals of*

Internal Medicine, 165(12):895–897, December 2016. URL: http://dx.doi.org/10.7326/L16-0534, doi:10.7326/l16-0534.

[95] Ethan A Litman, Steven L Gortmaker, Cara B Ebbeling, and David S Ludwig. Source of bias in sugar-sweetened beverage research: a systematic review. *Public Health Nutrition*, 21(12):2345–2350, March 2018. URL: http://dx.doi.org/10.1017/S1368980018000575, doi:10.1017/s1368980018000575.

[96] Marion Nestle. Food Lobbies, the Food Pyramid, and U.S. Nutrition Policy. *International Journal of Health Services*, 23(3):483–496, July 1993. URL: http://dx.doi.org/10.2190/32F2-2PFB-MEG7-8HPU, doi:10.2190/32f2-2pfb-meg7-8hpu.

[97] Mary T. Newport and Fabian M. Dayrit. The Lipid–Heart Hypothesis and the Keys Equation Defined the Dietary Guidelines but Ignored the Impact of Trans-Fat and High Linoleic Acid Consumption. *Nutrients*, 16(10):1447, May 2024. URL: http://dx.doi.org/10.3390/nu16101447, doi:10.3390/nu16101447.

[98] Nina Teicholz. A short history of saturated fat: the making and unmaking of a scientific consensus. *Current Opinion in Endocrinology, Diabetes & Obesity*, 30(1):65–71, December 2022. URL: http://dx.doi.org/10.1097/MED.0000000000000791, doi:10.1097/med.0000000000000791.

[99] Shailesh Nagpure, Kushagra Mathur, RajatKumar Agrawal, and Deepali Deshpande. Effect of artificial sweeteners on insulin resistance among type-2 diabetes mellitus patients. *Journal of Family Medicine and Primary Care*, 9(1):69, 2020. URL: http://dx.doi.org/10.4103/jfmpc.jfmpc_329_19, doi:10.4103/jfmpc.jfmpc_329_19.

[100] Michelle Pearlman, Jon Obert, and Lisa Casey. The Association Between Artificial Sweeteners and Obesity. *Current Gastroenterology Reports*, November 2017. URL: http://dx.doi.org/10.1007/s11894-017-0602-9, doi:10.1007/s11894-017-0602-9.

[101] Kiyah J Duffey, Lyn M Steffen, Linda Van Horn, Jr Jacobs, David R, and Barry M Popkin. Dietary patterns matter: diet beverages and cardiometabolic risks in the longitudinal Coronary Artery Risk Development in Young Adults (CARDIA) Study. *The American Journal of Clinical Nutrition*, 95(4):909–915, April 2012. URL: http://dx.doi.org/10.3945/ajcn.111.026682, doi:10.3945/ajcn.111.026682.

[102] Jeffrey L. Fortuna. Sweet Preference, Sugar Addiction and the Familial History of Alcohol Dependence: Shared Neural Pathways and Genes. *Journal of Psychoactive Drugs*, 42(2):147–151, June 2010. URL: http://dx.doi.org/10.1080/02791072.2010.10400687, doi:10.1080/02791072.2010.10400687.

[103] C. H. Wideman, G. R. Nadzam, and H. M. Murphy. Implications of an animal model of sugar addiction, withdrawal and relapse for human health. *Nutritional Neuroscience*, 8(5–6):269–276, October 2005. URL: http://dx.doi.org/10.1080/10284150500485221, doi:10.1080/10284150500485221.

[104] James J DiNicolantonio, James H O'Keefe, and William L Wilson. Sugar addiction: is it real? A narrative review. *British Journal of Sports Medicine*, 52(14):910–913, August 2017. URL: http://dx.doi.org/10.1136/bjsports-2017-097971, doi:10.1136/bjsports-2017-097971.

[105] Adrian Furnham and Hua Chu Boo. A literature review of the anchoring effect. *The Journal of Socio-Economics*, 40(1):35–42, February 2011. URL: http://dx.doi.org/10.1016/j.socec.2010.10.008, doi:10.1016/j.socec.2010.10.008.

[106] Susan B. Roberts. High-glycemic Index Foods, Hunger, and Obesity: Is There a Connection? *Nutrition Reviews*, 58(6):163–169, April 2009. URL: http://dx.doi.org/10.1111/j.1753-4887.2000.tb01855.x, doi:10.1111/j.1753-4887.2000.tb01855.x.

[107] Lee S Gross, Li Li, Earl S Ford, and Simin Liu. Increased consumption of refined carbohydrates and the epidemic of type 2 diabetes in the United States: an ecologic assessment. *The American Journal of Clinical Nutrition*, 79(5):774–779, May 2004. URL: http://dx.doi.o rg/10.1093/ajcn/79.5.774, doi:10.1093/ajcn/79.5.774.

[108] Amin Salehi Abargouei, Naser Kalantari, Nasrin Omidvar, Bahram Rashidkhani, Anahita Houshiar Rad, Azizeh Afkham Ebrahimi, Hossein Khosravi-Boroujeni, and Ahmad Esmaillzadeh. Refined carbohydrate intake in relation to non-verbal intelligence among Tehrani schoolchildren. *Public Health Nutrition*, 15(10):1925–1931, December 2011. URL: http://dx.doi.org/10.1017/S13689800110033 02, doi:10.1017/s1368980011003302.

[109] Ganesan Radhika, Rob M. Van Dam, Vasudevan Sudha, Anbazhagan Ganesan, and Viswanathan Mohan. Refined grain consumption and the metabolic syndrome in urban Asian Indians (Chennai Urban Rural Epidemiology Study 57). *Metabolism*, 58(5):675–681, May 2009. URL: http://dx.doi.org/10.1016/j.metabol.2009.01.008, doi:10.1016/j.metabol.2009.01.008.

[110] Hannah H. Tuson, Matthew H. Foley, Nicole M. Koropatkin, and Julie S. Biteen. The Starch Utilization System Assembles around Stationary Starch-Binding Proteins. *Biophysical Journal*, 115(2):242–250, July 2018. URL: http://dx.doi.org/10.1016/j.bpj.2017.12.015, doi:10.1016/j.bpj.2017.12.015.

[111] Harry J. Flint, Karen P. Scott, Sylvia H. Duncan, Petra Louis, and Evelyne Forano. Microbial degradation of complex carbohydrates in the gut. *Gut Microbes*, 3(4):289–306, May 2012. URL: http://dx.doi .org/10.4161/gmic.19897, doi:10.4161/gmic.19897.

[112] Kyu Hong Cho, Diedre Cho, Gui-Rong Wang, and Abigail A. Salyers. New Regulatory Gene That Contributes to Control of Bacteroides thetaiotaomicron Starch Utilization Genes. *Journal of Bacteriology*,

183(24):7198–7205, December 2001. URL: http://dx.doi.org/10.1128/JB.183.24.7198-7205.2001, doi:10.1128/jb.183.24.7198-7205.2001.

[113] Hannah M. Wexler. Bacteroides: the Good, the Bad, and the Nitty-Gritty. *Clinical Microbiology Reviews*, 20(4):593–621, October 2007. URL: http://dx.doi.org/10.1128/CMR.00008-07, doi:10.1128/cmr.00008-07.

[114] Alida CM Veloo, Kathleen E Boiten, Antoni PA Hendrickx, Joffrey van Prehn, and John WA Rossen. Horizontal gene transfer of a cfiA element between two different Bacteroides species within a clinical specimen. *Clinical Microbiology and Infection*, 30(4):554–555, 2024. URL: https://www.clinicalmicrobiologyandinfection.com/article/S1198-743X(23)00630-4/fulltext.

[115] Carlos Quesada-Gómez. Bacteroides mobilizable and conjugative genetic elements: antibiotic resistance among clinical isolates. *Revista Española de Quimioterapia*, 2011. URL: https://www.seq.es/seq/0214-3429/24/4/quesada.pdf.

[116] Kelly Louise Jobling. Horizontal gene transfer in Bacteroides fragilis. *Edinburgh Research Archive*, 2014. URL: https://era.ed.ac.uk/handle/1842/9637.

[117] William Jogia and Corinne F. Maurice. Polysaccharide Protection: How Bacteroides thetaiotaomicron Survives an Antibiotic Attack. *Cell Metabolism*, 30(4):619–621, October 2019. URL: http://dx.doi.org/10.1016/j.cmet.2019.09.011, doi:10.1016/j.cmet.2019.09.011.

[118] Yuqi Gao, Rui Hua, Kezheng Peng, Yuemiao Yin, Chenye Zeng, Yannan Guo, Yida Wang, Liyuan Li, Xue Li, Ying Qiu, and Zhao Wang. High-starchy carbohydrate diet aggravates NAFLD by increasing fatty acids influx mediated by NOX2. *Food Science and Human Wellness*, 12(4):1081–1101, July 2023. URL: http://dx.doi.org/10.1016/j.fshw.2022.10.026, doi:10.1016/j.fshw.2022.10.026.

[119] Jing Wang, LIjuan Huang, Hua Li, Guohong Chen, Liming Yang, Dong Wang, Hong Han, Guo Zheng, Xu Wang, Jianmin Liang, Weijie He, Fang Fang, Jianxiang Liao, and Dan Sun. Effects of ketogenic diet on the classification and functional composition of intestinal flora in children with mitochondrial epilepsy. *Frontiers in Neurology*, July 2023. URL: http://dx.doi.org/10.3389/fneur.2023.1237255, doi:10.3389/fneur.2023.1237255.

[120] B. Meding, K. Wrangsjö, J. Brisman, and B. Järvholm. Hand eczema in 45 bakers − a clinical study. *Contact Dermatitis*, 48(1):7–11, January 2003. URL: http://dx.doi.org/10.1034/j.1600-0536.2003 .480102.x, doi:10.1034/j.1600-0536.2003.480102.x.

[121] A Ivarsson, LÅ Persson, L Nyström, H Ascher, B Cavell, L Danielsson, A Dannaeus, T Lindberg, B Lindquist, L Stenhammar, and O Hernell. Epidemic of coeliac disease in Swedish children. *Acta Paediatrica*, 89(2):165–171, February 2000. URL: http://dx.doi.o rg/10.1111/j.1651-2227.2000.tb01210.x, doi:10.1111/j.1651-2227.2000.tb01210.x.

[122] Alberto Rubio–Tapia, Robert A. Kyle, Edward L. Kaplan, Dwight R. Johnson, William Page, Frederick Erdtmann, Tricia L. Brantner, W. Ray Kim, Tara K. Phelps, Brian D. Lahr, Alan R. Zinsmeister, III Melton, L. Joseph, and Joseph A. Murray. Increased Prevalence and Mortality in Undiagnosed Celiac Disease. *Gastroenterology*, 137(1):88–93, July 2009. URL: http://dx.doi.org/10.1053/j.gastro. 2009.03.059, doi:10.1053/j.gastro.2009.03.059.

[123] Anna Sapone, Julio C Bai, Carolina Ciacci, Jernej Dolinsek, Peter HR Green, Marios Hadjivassiliou, Katri Kaukinen, Kamran Rostami, David S Sanders, Michael Schumann, Reiner Ullrich, Danilo Villalta, Umberto Volta, Carlo Catassi, and Alessio Fasano. Spectrum of gluten-related disorders: consensus on new nomenclature and classification. *BMC Medicine*, February 2012. URL: http://dx.doi.org/10.1186/174 1-7015-10-13, doi:10.1186/1741-7015-10-13.

[124] Torsten Matthias, Sandra Neidhöfer, Sascha Pfeiffer, Kai Prager, Sandra Reuter, and M Eric Gershwin. Novel trends in celiac disease. *Cellular & Molecular Immunology*, 8(2):121–125, January 2011. URL: http://dx.doi.org/10.1038/cmi.2010.68, doi:10.1038/cmi.2010.68.

[125] Hetty C. van den Broeck, Hein C. de Jong, Elma M. J. Salentijn, Liesbeth Dekking, Dirk Bosch, Rob J. Hamer, Ludovicus J. W. J. Gilissen, Ingrid M. van der Meer, and Marinus J. M. Smulders. Presence of celiac disease epitopes in modern and old hexaploid wheat varieties: wheat breeding may have contributed to increased prevalence of celiac disease. *Theoretical and Applied Genetics*, 121(8):1527–1539, July 2010. URL: http://dx.doi.org/10.1007/s00 122-010-1408-4, doi:10.1007/s00122-010-1408-4.

[126] R Baird Shuman. Borlaug receives The nobel prize for his work on World hunger: EBSCO. 2023. URL: https://www.ebsco.com/resear ch-starters/economics/borlaug-receives-nobel-prize-his-work-world -hunger.

[127] Aug 2022. URL: https://resource.rockarch.org/story/the-rockefeller-f oundations-mexican-agriculture-program-1943-1965/.

[128] Thomas A Lumpkin. How a gene from Japan revolutionized the world of wheat: CIMMYT's quest for combining genes to mitigate threats to global food security. In *Advances in wheat genetics: From genome to field: Proceedings of the 12th International Wheat Genetics Symposium*, 13–20. Springer Japan, 2015. URL: https://link.springer. com/chapter/10.1007/978-4-431-55675-6_2.

[129] José María Remes-Troche, Aurelio Rios-Vaca, María Teresa Ramírez-Iglesias, Alberto Rubio-Tapia, Vicente Andrade-Zarate, Fanny Rodríguez-Vallejo, Francisco López-Maldonado, Francisco Javier Gomez-Perez, and Luis F. Uscanga. High Prevalence of Celiac Disease in Mexican Mestizo Adults With Type 1 Diabetes Mellitus.

Journal of Clinical Gastroenterology, 42(5):460–465, May 2008. URL: http://dx.doi.org/10.1097/MCG.0b013e318046ea86, doi:10.1097/mcg.0b013e318046ea86.

[130] Bernardo Turnbull, Sarah Frances Gordon, Gloria Oliva Martínez-Andrade, and Marco González-Unzaga. Childhood obesity in Mexico: A critical analysis of the environmental factors, behaviours and discourses contributing to the epidemic. *Health Psychology Open*, January 2019. URL: http://dx.doi.org/10.1177/2055102919849406, doi:10.1177/2055102919849406.

[131] Jesús-Daniel Zazueta-Borboa, Rafael Samper-Ternent, Rebeca Wong, and Neil Mehta. Economic Disadvantage During Childhood, Obesity, and Diabetes Across Three Birth Cohorts of Older Mexicans. *The Journals of Gerontology, Series B: Psychological Sciences and Social Sciences*, October 2024. URL: http://dx.doi.org/10.1093/geronb/gbae178, doi:10.1093/geronb/gbae178.

[132] Ming-Sheng Fan, Fang-Jie Zhao, Susan J. Fairweather-Tait, Paul R. Poulton, Sarah J. Dunham, and Steve P. McGrath. Evidence of decreasing mineral density in wheat grain over the last 160 years. *Journal of Trace Elements in Medicine and Biology*, 22(4):315–324, November 2008. URL: http://dx.doi.org/10.1016/j.jtemb.2008.07.002, doi:10.1016/j.jtemb.2008.07.002.

[133] Norman Temple. Fat, Sugar, Whole Grains and Heart Disease: 50 Years of Confusion. *Nutrients*, 10(1):39, January 2018. URL: http://dx.doi.org/10.3390/nu10010039, doi:10.3390/nu10010039.

[134] Monika A. Gorzelak, Amanda K. Asay, Brian J. Pickles, and Suzanne W. Simard. Inter-plant communication through mycorrhizal networks mediates complex adaptive behaviour in plant communities. *AoB Plants*, 7:plv050, 2015. URL: http://dx.doi.org/10.1093/aobpla/plv050, doi:10.1093/aobpla/plv050.

[135] Julia Dordel and Guido Tölke. The Hidden Language of Trees: How Forests Secretly Communicate | Full documentary.

[136] Taylor C. Wallace. A Comprehensive Review of Eggs, Choline, and Lutein on Cognition Across the Life-span. *Journal of the American College of Nutrition*, 37(4):269–285, February 2018. URL: http://dx.doi.org/10.1080/07315724.2017.1423248, doi:10.1080/07315724.2017.1423248.

[137] Soyogu Yamashita, Naoki Kawada, Wei Wang, Kenta Susaki, Yumi Takeda, Mamoru Kimura, Yoshitaka Iwama, Yutaka Miura, Michihiro Sugano, and Ryosuke Matsuoka. Effects of egg yolk choline intake on cognitive functions and plasma choline levels in healthy middle-aged and older Japanese: a randomized double-blinded placebo-controlled parallel-group study. *Lipids in Health and Disease*, June 2023. URL: http://dx.doi.org/10.1186/s12944-023-01844-w, doi:10.1186/s12944-023-01844-w.

[138] Michael J. Puglisi and Maria Luz Fernandez. The Health Benefits of Egg Protein. *Nutrients*, 14(14):2904, July 2022. URL: http://dx.doi.org/10.3390/nu14142904, doi:10.3390/nu14142904.

[139] Jennifer Kovacs-Nolan, Marshall Phillips, and Yoshinori Mine. Advances in the Value of Eggs and Egg Components for Human Health. *Journal of Agricultural and Food Chemistry*, 53(22):8421–8431, September 2005. URL: http://dx.doi.org/10.1021/jf050964f, doi:10.1021/jf050964f.

[140] Gisella Mutungi, Joseph Ratliff, Michael Puglisi, Moises Torres-Gonzalez, Ushma Vaishnav, Jose O. Leite, Erin Quann, Jeff S. Volek, and Maria Luz Fernandez. Dietary Cholesterol from Eggs Increases Plasma HDL Cholesterol in Overweight Men Consuming a Carbohydrate-Restricted Diet ,2. *The Journal of Nutrition*, 138(2):272–276, February 2008. URL: http://dx.doi.org/10.1093/jn/138.2.272, doi:10.1093/jn/138.2.272.

[141] Walter L. Miller. Steroid hormone synthesis in mitochondria. *Molecular and Cellular Endocrinology*, 379(1–2):62–73, October 2013. URL: http://dx.doi.org/10.1016/j.mce.2013.04.014, doi:10.1016/j.mce.2013.04.014.

[142] Agnieszka Latoch, Dariusz Mirosław Stasiak, and Patryk Siczek. Edible Offal as a Valuable Source of Nutrients in the Diet—A Review. *Nutrients*, 16(11):1609, May 2024. URL: http://dx.doi.org/10.3390/nu16111609, doi:10.3390/nu16111609.

[143] Beef, variety meats and by-products, liver, cooked, braised. URL: https://fdc.nal.usda.gov/food-details/168626/nutrients.

[144] Rui Zhang, Huai Zhang, Yi Wang, Liang-Jie Tang, Gang Li, Ou-Yang Huang, Sui-Dan Chen, Giovanni Targher, Christopher D. Byrne, Bin-Bin Gu, and Ming-Hua Zheng. Higher consumption of animal organ meat is associated with a lower prevalence of nonalcoholic steatohepatitis. *Hepatobiliary Surgery and Nutrition*, 12(5):645–657, October 2023. URL: http://dx.doi.org/10.21037/hbsn-21-468, doi:10.21037/hbsn-21-468.

[145] Juana P. Díaz-Alarcón, Miguel Navarro-Alarcón, Herminia López-García de la Serrana, and María C. López-Martínez. Determination of Selenium in Meat Products by Hydride Generation Atomic Absorption SpectrometrySelenium Levels in Meat, Organ Meats, and Sausages in Spain. *Journal of Agricultural and Food Chemistry*, 44(6):1494–1497, January 1996. URL: http://dx.doi.org/10.1021/jf950702l, doi:10.1021/jf950702l.

[146] Paweł Gać, Karolina Czerwińska, Piotr Macek, Aleksandra Jaremków, Grzegorz Mazur, Krystyna Pawlas, and Rafał Poręba. The importance of selenium and zinc deficiency in cardiovascular disorders. *Environmental Toxicology and Pharmacology*, 82:103553, February 2021. URL: http://dx.doi.org/10.1016/j.etap.2020.103553, doi:10.1016/j.etap.2020.103553.

[147] L.Y. Sun, F.G. Meng, Q. Li, Z.J. Zhao, C.Z. He, S.P. Wang, R.L. Sa, W.W. Man, and L.H. Wang. Effects of the consumption of rice from non-KBD areas and selenium supplementation on the prevention and treatment of paediatric Kaschin–Beck disease: an epidemiological intervention trial in the Qinghai Province. *Osteoarthritis and Cartilage*, 22(12):2033–2040, December 2014. URL: http://dx.doi.org/10.1016/j.joca.2014.09.013, doi:10.1016/j.joca.2014.09.013.

[148] Katarina M. Doma, Marc Moulin, Huda Al-Wahsh, Najla Guthrie, David C. Crowley, and Erin D. Lewis. An open-label clinical trial to investigate the safety and efficacy of a bone broth diet on weight loss in adults with obesity. *Clinical Nutrition Open Science*, 61:282–296, June 2025. URL: http://dx.doi.org/10.1016/j.nutos.2025.04.009, doi:10.1016/j.nutos.2025.04.009.

[149] Lifeng Wang, Fu-Sheng Wang, and M. Eric Gershwin. Human autoimmune diseases: a comprehensive update. *Journal of Internal Medicine*, 278(4):369–395, July 2015. URL: http://dx.doi.org/10.1111/joim.12395, doi:10.1111/joim.12395.

[150] Dimitrios P. Bogdanos, Daniel S. Smyk, Eirini I. Rigopoulou, Maria G. Mytilinaiou, Michael A. Heneghan, Carlo Selmi, and M. Eric Gershwin. Twin studies in autoimmune disease: Genetics, gender and environment. *Journal of Autoimmunity*, 38(2–3):J156–J169, May 2012. URL: http://dx.doi.org/10.1016/j.jaut.2011.11.003, doi:10.1016/j.jaut.2011.11.003.

[151] H. Bierne, M. Hamon, and P. Cossart. Epigenetics and Bacterial Infections. *Cold Spring Harbor Perspectives in Medicine*, 2(12):a010272–a010272, December 2012. URL: http://dx.doi.org/10.1101/cshperspect.a010272, doi:10.1101/cshperspect.a010272.

[152] María A. Sánchez-Romero and Josep Casadesús. The bacterial epigenome. *Nature Reviews Microbiology*, 18(1):7–20, November

2019. URL: http://dx.doi.org/10.1038/s41579-019-0286-2, doi:10.1038/s41579-019-0286-2.

[153] Jawara Allen, Stephanie Hao, Cynthia L. Sears, and Winston Timp. Epigenetic Changes Induced by Bacteroides fragilis Toxin. *Infection and Immunity*, June 2019. URL: http://dx.doi.org/10.1128/iai.00447 -18, doi:10.1128/iai.00447-18.

[154] Josep Casadesús and David Low. Epigenetic Gene Regulation in the Bacterial World. *Microbiology and Molecular Biology Reviews*, 70(3):830–856, September 2006. URL: http://dx.doi.org/10.1128/m mbr.00016-06, doi:10.1128/mmbr.00016-06.

[155] Alessio Fasano. Zonulin and Its Regulation of Intestinal Barrier Function: The Biological Door to Inflammation, Autoimmunity, and Cancer. *Physiological Reviews*, 91(1):151–175, January 2011. URL: http://dx.doi.org/10.1152/physrev.00003.2008, doi:10.1152/physrev.00003.2008.

[156] Feb 2024. URL: https://www.mcgill.ca/oss/article/medical-critical-t hinking/you-probably-dont-have-leaky-gut.

[157] Feb 2024. URL: https://badgut.org/information-centre/a-z-digestive -topics/leaky-gut-syndrome/.

[158] Yusuke Kinashi and Koji Hase. Partners in Leaky Gut Syndrome: Intestinal Dysbiosis and Autoimmunity. *Frontiers in Immunology*, April 2021. URL: http://dx.doi.org/10.3389/fimmu.2021.673708, doi:10.3389/fimmu.2021.673708.

[159] Alessio Fasano. Physiological, Pathological, and Therapeutic Implications of Zonulin-Mediated Intestinal Barrier Modulation. *The American Journal of Pathology*, 173(5):1243–1252, November 2008. URL: http://dx.doi.org/10.2353/ajpath.2008.080192, doi:10.2353/ajpath.2008.080192.

[160] Alessio Fasano. Leaky Gut and Autoimmune Diseases. *Clinical Reviews in Allergy & Immunology*, 42(1):71–78, November 2011. URL: http://dx.doi.org/10.1007/s12016-011-8291-x, doi:10.1007/s12016-011-8291-x.

[161] Bradley Leech, Janet Schloss, and Amie Steel. Treatment Interventions for the Management of Intestinal Permeability: A Cross-Sectional Survey of Complementary and Integrative Medicine Practitioners. *The Journal of Alternative and Complementary Medicine*, 25(6):623–636, June 2019. URL: http://dx.doi.org/10.1089/acm.2018.0374, doi:10.1089/acm.2018.0374.

[162] Stephan C Bischoff, Giovanni Barbara, Wim Buurman, Theo Ockhuizen, Jörg-Dieter Schulzke, Matteo Serino, Herbert Tilg, Alastair Watson, and Jerry M Wells. Intestinal permeability – a new target for disease prevention and therapy. *BMC Gastroenterology*, November 2014. URL: http://dx.doi.org/10.1186/s12876-014-018 9-7, doi:10.1186/s12876-014-0189-7.

[163] Yun Kit Yeoh, Tao Zuo, Grace Chung-Yan Lui, Fen Zhang, Qin Liu, Amy YL Li, Arthur CK Chung, Chun Pan Cheung, Eugene YK Tso, Kitty SC Fung, Veronica Chan, Lowell Ling, Gavin Joynt, David Shu-Cheong Hui, Kai Ming Chow, Susanna So Shan Ng, Timothy Chun-Man Li, Rita WY Ng, Terry CF Yip, Grace Lai-Hung Wong, Francis KL Chan, Chun Kwok Wong, Paul KS Chan, and Siew C Ng. Gut microbiota composition reflects disease severity and dysfunctional immune responses in patients with COVID-19. *Gut*, 70(4):698–706, January 2021. URL: http://dx.doi.org/10.1136/gut jnl-2020-323020, doi:10.1136/gutjnl-2020-323020.

[164] Zhonghan Sun, Zhi-Gang Song, Chenglin Liu, Shishang Tan, Shuchun Lin, Jiajun Zhu, Fa-Hui Dai, Jian Gao, Jia-Lei She, Zhendong Mei, Tao Lou, Jiao-Jiao Zheng, Yi Liu, Jiang He, Yuanting Zheng, Chen Ding, Feng Qian, Yan Zheng, and Yan-Mei Chen. Gut microbiome alterations and gut barrier dysfunction are associated with host

immune homeostasis in COVID-19 patients. *BMC Medicine*, January 2022. URL: http://dx.doi.org/10.1186/s12916-021-02212-0, doi:10.1186/s12916-021-02212-0.

[165] Ayah Matar, Nada Abdelnaem, and Michael Camilleri. Bone Broth Benefits: How Its Nutrients Fortify Gut Barrier in Health and Disease. *Digestive Diseases and Sciences*, April 2025. URL: http://dx.doi.org /10.1007/s10620-025-08997-x, doi:10.1007/s10620-025-08997-x.

[166] Jason Hannan. "But Bacon!" The Performative Violence of Anti-Vegan Trolling 1. In *Violence and Harm in the Animal Industrial Complex*, pages 54–68. Routledge, 2024. URL: https://www.taylor francis.com/chapters/edit/10.4324/9781003441908-5/bacon-perform ative-violence-anti-vegan-trolling-1-jason-hannan.

[167] Joshua Doyle and Alex Richardson. The moderating role of post-materialism in the relationship between income and red meat consumption. *International Journal of Sociology*, pages 1–19, March 2025. URL: http://dx.doi.org/10.1080/00207659.2025.2473207, doi:10.1080/00207659.2025.2473207.

[168] S. Marek Muller, David Rooney, and Cecilia Cerja. Long live the Liver King: right-wing carnivorism and the digital dissemination of primal rhetoric. *Frontiers in Communication*, March 2024. URL: http://dx.doi.org/10.3389/fcomm.2024.1338653, doi:10.3389/fcomm.2024.1338653.

[169] Doyeon Kim and Yongsoon Park. Amount of Protein Required to Improve Muscle Mass in Older Adults. *Nutrients*, 12(6):1700, June 2020. URL: http://dx.doi.org/10.3390/nu12061700, doi:10.3390/nu12061700.

[170] Tim Noakes and Nutrition Network. The Ancel Keys Cholesterol Con. Part 12. 1984-1993. *The Noakes Foundation*, sep 2023. URL: https://thenoakesfoundation.org/the-ancel-keys-cholesterol-con-part-12-1 984-1993/.

[171] Ghada A. Soliman. Dietary Cholesterol and the Lack of Evidence in Cardiovascular Disease. *Nutrients*, 10(6):780, June 2018. URL: http://dx.doi.org/10.3390/nu10060780, doi:10.3390/nu10060780.

[172] Arne Astrup, Faidon Magkos, Dennis M. Bier, J. Thomas Brenna, Marcia C. de Oliveira Otto, James O. Hill, Janet C. King, Andrew Mente, Jose M. Ordovas, Jeff S. Volek, Salim Yusuf, and Ronald M. Krauss. Saturated Fats and Health: A Reassessment and Proposal for Food-Based Recommendations. *Journal of the American College of Cardiology*, 76(7):844–857, August 2020. URL: http://dx.doi.org/10.1016/j.jacc.2020.05.077, doi:10.1016/j.jacc.2020.05.077.

[173] David M Goldman, Thomas J Waterfall, and Matthew Nagra. Traditional Maasai Dietary Practices and Their Inapplicability to Modern Carnivore Diets: A Narrative Review. *Cureus*, February 2025. URL: http://dx.doi.org/10.7759/cureus.78448, doi:10.7759/cureus.78448.

[174] Jaecheol Moon and Gwanpyo Koh. Clinical Evidence and Mechanisms of High-Protein Diet-Induced Weight Loss. *Journal of Obesity & Metabolic Syndrome*, 29(3):166–173, September 2020. URL: http://dx.doi.org/10.7570/jomes20028, doi:10.7570/jomes20028.

[175] Ulrike Haß, Sarah Heider, Bastian Kochlik, Catrin Herpich, Olga Pivovarova-Ramich, and Kristina Norman. Effects of Exercise and Omega-3-Supplemented, High-Protein Diet on Inflammatory Markers in Serum, on Gene Expression Levels in PBMC, and after Ex Vivo Whole-Blood LPS Stimulation in Old Adults. *International Journal of Molecular Sciences*, 24(2):928, January 2023. URL: http://dx.doi.org/10.3390/ijms24020928, doi:10.3390/ijms24020928.

[176] Michael J. Macartney, Mathew M. Ghodsian, Bransen Noel-Gough, Peter L. McLennan, and Gregory E. Peoples. DHA-Rich Fish Oil Increases the Omega-3 Index in Healthy Adults and Slows Resting

Heart Rate without Altering Cardiac Autonomic Reflex Modulation. *Journal of the American Nutrition Association*, 41(7):637–645, August 2021. URL: http://dx.doi.org/10.1080/07315724.2021.1953417, doi:10.1080/07315724.2021.1953417.

[177] Nicholas J. Sjoberg, Catherine M. Milte, Jonathan D. Buckley, Peter R. C. Howe, Alison M. Coates, and David A. Saint. Dose-dependent increases in heart rate variability and arterial compliance in overweight and obese adults with DHA-rich fish oil supplementation. *British Journal of Nutrition*, 103(2):243–248, August 2009. URL: http://dx.doi.org/10.1017/S000711450999153X, doi:10.1017/s000711450999153x.

[178] Peter L. McLennan. Cardiac physiology and clinical efficacy of dietary fish oil clarified through cellular mechanisms of omega-3 polyunsaturated fatty acids. *European Journal of Applied Physiology*, 114(7):1333–1356, April 2014. URL: http://dx.doi.org/10.1007/s00421-014-2876-z, doi:10.1007/s00421-014-2876-z.

[179] Feb 2021. URL: https://www.hcplive.com/view/fish-oil-supplements-may-lower-cardiac-risk--by-increasing-heart-rate-variability.

[180] Lauren A Stahl, Denovan P Begg, Richard S Weisinger, and Andrew J Sinclair. The role of omega-3 fatty acids in mood disorders. *Current Opinion in Investigational Drugs*, 9(1):57–64, 2008. URL: https://www.researchgate.net/publication/5665970_The_role_of_omega-3_fatty_acids_in_mood_disorders.

[181] Kayla R. Zehr and Mary K. Walker. Omega-3 polyunsaturated fatty acids improve endothelial function in humans at risk for atherosclerosis: A review. *Prostaglandins & Other Lipid Mediators*, 134:131–140, January 2018. URL: http://dx.doi.org/10.1016/j.prostaglandins.2017.07.005, doi:10.1016/j.prostaglandins.2017.07.005.

[182] Pitchai Balakumar and Gaurav Taneja. Fish oil and vascular endothelial protection: Bench to bedside. *Free Radical Biology and Medicine*, 53(2):271–279, July 2012. URL: h t tp : / / d x . d o i . o r g / 1 0 . 1 0 1 6 / j . f r e e r a d b i o m e d . 2 0 1 2 . 0 5 . 0 05, doi:10.1016/j.freeradbiomed.2012.05.005.

[183] Mahsa Elahikhah, Fatemeh Haidari, Saman Khalesi, Hajieh Shahbazian, Majid Mohammadshahi, and Vahideh Aghamohammadi. Milk protein concentrate supplementation improved appetite, metabolic parameters, adipocytokines, and body composition in dieting women with obesity: a randomized controlled trial. *BMC Nutrition*, June 2024. URL: http://dx.doi.org/10.1186/s40795-024-0 0879-1, doi:10.1186/s40795-024-00879-1.

[184] Jo-Anne Gilbert, Denis R. Joanisse, Jean-Philippe Chaput, Pierre Miegueu, Katherine Cianflone, Natalie Alméras, and Angelo Tremblay. Milk supplementation facilitates appetite control in obese women during weight loss: a randomised, single-blind, placebo-controlled trial. *British Journal of Nutrition*, 105(1):133–143, December 2010. URL: http://dx.doi.org/10.1017/S00071145100031 19, doi:10.1017/s0007114510003119.

[185] Kênia M. B. de Carvalho, Nathalia Pizato, Patrícia B. Botelho, Eliane S. Dutra, and Vivian S. S. Gonçalves. Dietary protein and appetite sensations in individuals with overweight and obesity: a systematic review. *European Journal of Nutrition*, 59(6):2317–2332, July 2020. URL: http://dx.doi.org/10.1007/s00394-020-02321-1, doi:10.1007/s00394-020-02321-1.

[186] B. Kung, G.H. Anderson, S. Paré, A.J. Tucker, S. Vien, A.J. Wright, and H.D. Goff. Effect of milk protein intake and casein-to-whey ratio in breakfast meals on postprandial glucose, satiety ratings, and subsequent meal intake. *Journal of Dairy Science*, 101(10):8688–8701, October 2018. URL: http://dx.doi.org/10.3168/jds.2018-14419, doi:10.3168/jds.2018-14419.

[187] L.B. Dalgaard, D.Z. Kruse, K. Norup, B.V. Andersen, and M. Hansen. A dairy-based, protein-rich breakfast enhances satiety and cognitive concentration before lunch in overweight to obese young females: A randomized controlled crossover study. *Journal of Dairy Science*, 107(5):2653–2667, May 2024. URL: http://dx.doi.org/10.3168/jds.2 023-24152, doi:10.3168/jds.2023-24152.

[188] Gang Tang, Wang Huang, Jie Tao, and Zhengqiang Wei. Prophylactic effects of probiotics or synbiotics on postoperative ileus after gastrointestinal cancer surgery: A meta-analysis of randomized controlled trials. *PLOS ONE*, 17(3):e0264759, March 2022. URL: http://dx.doi.org/10.1371/journal.pone.0264759, doi:10.1371/journal.pone.0264759.

[189] Z. Liu, H. Qin, Z. Yang, Y. Xia, W. Liu, J. Yang, Y. Jiang, H. Zhang, Z. Yang, Y. Wang, and Q. Zheng. Randomised clinical trial: the effects of perioperative probiotic treatment on barrier function and post-operative infectious complications in colorectal cancer surgery – a double-blind study. *Alimentary Pharmacology & Therapeutics*, 33(1):50–63, October 2010. URL: http://dx.doi.org/10.1111/j.1365-2 036.2010.04492.x, doi:10.1111/j.1365-2036.2010.04492.x.

[190] Yingzi Yuan, Yutong Yang, Lele Xiao, Lingbo Qu, Xiaoling Zhang, and Yongjun Wei. Advancing Insights into Probiotics during Vegetable Fermentation. *Foods*, 12(20):3789, October 2023. URL: http://dx.doi.org/10.3390/foods12203789, doi:10.3390/foods12203789.

[191] Thilakna Ampemohotti, Aida Golneshin, Christopher Pillidge, Charles Brennan, and Thi Thu Hao Van. Fermented Vegetables: Their Microbiology and Impact on Gut Microbiota and Overall Health Benefits. *Food Reviews International*, pages 1–24, April 2025. URL: http://dx.doi.org/10.1080/87559129.2025.2486274, doi:10.1080/87559129.2025.2486274.

[192] Eman Shawky, Shelini Surendran, and Rasha M. Abu El-Khair. Fermented Vegetables as a Source of Psychobiotics: A Review of the Evidence for Mental Health Benefits. *Probiotics and Antimicrobial Proteins*, May 2025. URL: http://dx.doi.org/10.1007/s12602-025-1 0592-5, doi:10.1007/s12602-025-10592-5.

[193] Lei Wei and Maria L. Marco. The fermented cabbage metabolome and its protection against cytokine-induced intestinal barrier disruption of Caco-2 monolayers. *Applied and Environmental Microbiology*, May 2025. URL: http://dx.doi.org/10.1128/aem.02234-24, doi:10.1128/aem.02234-24.

[194] Eduardo A.F. Nilson, Felipe Mendes Delpino, Carolina Batis, Priscila Pereira Machado, Jean-Claude Moubarac, Gustavo Cediel, Camila Corvalan, Gerson Ferrari, Fernanda Rauber, Euridice Martinez-Steele, Maria Laura da Costa Louzada, Renata Bertazzi Levy, Carlos A. Monteiro, and Leandro F.M. Rezende. Premature Mortality Attributable to Ultraprocessed Food Consumption in 8 Countries. *American Journal of Preventive Medicine*, 68(6):1091–1099, June 2025. URL: http://dx.doi.org/10.1016/j.amepre.2025 .02.018, doi:10.1016/j.amepre.2025.02.018.

[195] Haiyue Ren, Feng Zhao, Qiqi Zhang, Xing Huang, and Zhe Wang. Autophagy and skin wound healing. *Burns & Trauma*, January 2022. URL: http://dx.doi.org/10.1093/burnst/tkac003, doi:10.1093/burnst/tkac003.

[196] Isei Tanida. Autophagy basics. *Microbiology and Immunology*, 55(1):1–11, December 2010. URL: http://dx.doi.org/10.1111/j.134 8-0421.2010.00271.x, doi:10.1111/j.1348-0421.2010.00271.x.

[197] The Nobel Prize in Physiology or Medicine 2016, year=2016, month=Oct. URL: https://www.nobelprize.org/prizes/medicine/2 016/press-release/.

[198] Harald Renz. Autophagy: Nobel Prize 2016 and allergy and asthma research. *Journal of Allergy and Clinical Immunology*, 140(6):1548–1549, December 2017. URL: http://dx.doi.org/10.1016/j.jaci.2017.03.021, doi:10.1016/j.jaci.2017.03.021.

[199] Katherine K. Clifton, Cynthia X. Ma, Luigi Fontana, and Lindsay L. Peterson. Intermittent fasting in the prevention and treatment of cancer. *CA: A Cancer Journal for Clinicians*, 71(6):527–546, August 2021. URL: http://dx.doi.org/10.3322/caac.21694, doi:10.3322/caac.21694.

[200] Amandine Chaix, Emily N.C. Manoogian, Girish C. Melkani, and Satchidananda Panda. Time-Restricted Eating to Prevent and Manage Chronic Metabolic Diseases. *Annual Review of Nutrition*, 39(1):291–315, August 2019. URL: http://dx.doi.org/10.1146/annurev-nutr-082018-124320, doi:10.1146/annurev-nutr-082018-124320.

[201] Anita Choudhary, Bhagyashri Chakole, Ajay Kumar Yadav, Mahesh Vyas, and Meera K. Bhojani. An effect of one meal a day among the patients with Medo Dushti (dyslipidemia): a case series. *Journal of Indian System of Medicine*, 12(1):25–31, January 2024. URL: http://dx.doi.org/10.4103/jism.jism_70_23, doi:10.4103/jism.jism_70_23.

[202] Tam Pham, Zen Juen Lau, S. H. Annabel Chen, and Dominique Makowski. Heart Rate Variability in Psychology: A Review of HRV Indices and an Analysis Tutorial. *Sensors*, 21(12):3998, June 2021. URL: http://dx.doi.org/10.3390/s21123998, doi:10.3390/s21123998.

[203] Aiyong Cui, Tiansong Zhang, Peilong Xiao, Zhiqiang Fan, Hu Wang, and Yan Zhuang. Global and regional prevalence of vitamin D deficiency in population-based studies from 2000 to 2022: A pooled analysis of 7.9 million participants. *Frontiers in Nutrition*, Mar 2023. doi:10.3389/fnut.2023.1070808.

[204] Pawel Pludowski, Michael F. Holick, William B. Grant, Jerzy Konstantynowicz, Mario R. Mascarenhas, Afrozul Haq, Vladyslav Povoroznyuk, Nataliya Balatska, Ana Paula Barbosa, Tatiana

Karonova, Ema Rudenka, Waldemar Misiorowski, Irina Zakharova, Alena Rudenka, Jacek Łukaszkiewicz, Ewa Marcinowska-Suchowierska, Natalia Łaszcz, Pawel Abramowicz, Harjit P. Bhattoa, and Sunil J. Wimalawansa. Vitamin D supplementation guidelines. *The Journal of Steroid Biochemistry and Molecular Biology*, 175:125–135, 2018. Vitamin D Deficiency and Human Health. URL: https://www.sciencedirect.com/science/article/pii/S0960076017300316, doi:https://doi.org/10.1016/j.jsbmb.2017.01.021.

[205] Pawel Pludowski, William B. Grant, Spyridon N. Karras, Armin Zittermann, and Stefan Pilz. Vitamin D Supplementation: A Review of the Evidence Arguing for a Daily Dose of 2000 International Units (50 μg) of Vitamin D for Adults in the General Population. *Nutrients*, 2024. URL: https://www.mdpi.com/2072-6643/16/3/391, doi:10.3390/nu16030391.

[206] S. M. Kimball, N. Mirhosseini, and M. F. Holick and. Evaluation of vitamin D3 intakes up to 15,000 international units/day and serum 25-hydroxyvitamin D concentrations up to 300 nmol/L on calcium metabolism in a community setting. *Dermato-Endocrinology*, 9(1):e1300213, 2017. PMID: 28458767. URL: https://doi.org/10.1080/19381980.2017.1300213, arXiv:https://doi.org/10.1080/19381980.2017.1300213, doi:10.1080/19381980.2017.1300213.

[207] C N H Long. The Endocrine Control of the Blood Sugar. *Diabetes*, 1(1):3–11, January 1952. URL: http://dx.doi.org/10.2337/diab.1.1.3, doi:10.2337/diab.1.1.3.

[208] Taira Kajisa. Adrenaline rush in athletes: Visualizing glucose fluctuations during high-intensity races. 2023. URL: https://figshare.com/articles/dataset/_strong_Adrenaline_rush_in_athletes_Visualizing_glucose_fluctuations_during_high-intensity_races_strong_/22807130, doi:10.6084/M9.FIGSHARE.22807130.

[209] Meldijana Omerbegović, Amira Durić, Nusreta Muratović, Lejla Mulalić, and Emina Hamzanija. [Metabolic response to trauma and stress]. *Medicinski arhiv*, 57(4 Suppl 1):57—60, 2003. URL: http://europepmc.org/abstract/MED/15017867.

[210] M W Miller and N Sadeh. Traumatic stress, oxidative stress and post-traumatic stress disorder: neurodegeneration and the accelerated-aging hypothesis. *Molecular Psychiatry*, 19(11):1156–1162, September 2014. URL: http://dx.doi.org/10.1038/mp.2014.111, doi:10.1038/mp.2014.111.

[211] EM Peters, R Anderson, DC Nieman, H Fickl, and V Jogessar. Vitamin C supplementation attenuates the increases in circulating cortisol, adrenaline and anti-inflammatory polypeptides following ultramarathon running. *International journal of sports medicine*, 22(07):537–543, 2001. URL: https://www.thieme-connect.com/products/ejournals/abstract/10.1055/s-2001-17610.

[212] Srikumaran Melethil, William D. Mason, and Chang Chian-Jo. Dose-dependent absorption and excretion of vitamin C in humans. *International Journal of Pharmaceutics*, 31(1):83–89, 1986. URL: https://www.sciencedirect.com/science/article/pii/0378517386902164, doi:https://doi.org/10.1016/0378-5173(86)90216-4.

[213] Office of dietary supplements - vitamin C. URL: https://ods.od.nih.gov/factsheets/VitaminC-HealthProfessional/.

[214] Sreerag Gopi and Preetha Balakrishnan and. Evaluation and clinical comparison studies on liposomal and non-liposomal ascorbic acid (vitamin C) and their enhanced bioavailability. *Journal of Liposome Research*, 31(4):356–364, 2021. PMID: 32901526. URL: https://doi.org/10.1080/08982104.2020.1820521, arXiv:https://doi.org/10.1080/08982104.2020.1820521, doi:10.1080/08982104.2020.1820521.

[215] Stephen Hickey, Hilary J. Roberts, and Nicholas J. Miller and. Pharmacokinetics of oral vitamin C. *Journal of Nutritional & Environmental Medicine*, 17(3):169–177, 2008. URL: https://doi.org/10.1080/135908408023 0 5 4 2 3, arXiv:https://doi.org/10.1080/13590840802305423, doi:10.1080/13590840802305423.

[216] Martin Doseděl, Eduard Jirkovský, Kateřina Macáková, Lenka Krčmová, Lenka Javorská, Jana Pourová, Laura Mercolini, Fernando Remião, Lucie Nováková, and Přemysl Mladěnka. Vitamin C— Sources, Physiological Role, Kinetics, Deficiency, Use, Toxicity, and Determination. *Nutrients*, 13(2):615, February 2021. URL: http://dx .doi.org/10.3390/nu13020615, doi:10.3390/nu13020615.

[217] Christos T. Chasapis, Ariadni C. Loutsidou, Chara A. Spiliopoulou, and Maria E. Stefanidou. Zinc and human health: an update. *Archives of toxicology*, 86(4):521–534, 2012. doi:10.1007/s00204-011-0775-1.

[218] Paola Bonaventura, Giulia Benedetti, Francis Albarède, and Pierre Miossec. Zinc and its role in immunity and inflammation. *Autoimmunity Reviews*, 14(4):277–285, 2015. URL: https: //www.sciencedirect.com/science/article/pii/S1568997214002808, doi:https://doi.org/10.1016/j.autrev.2014.11.008.

[219] Maria Consolata Miletta, Martin H. Schöni, Kristin Kernland, Primus E. Mullis, and Vibor Petkovic. The role of zinc dynamics in growth hormone secretion. *Hormone Research in Paediatrics*, 80(6):381–389, 2013. doi:10.1159/000355408.

[220] Zhe Li, Yang Liu, Ruixue Wei, V. Wee Yong, and Mengzhou Xue. The Important Role of Zinc in Neurological Diseases. *Biomolecules*, 2023. URL: https://www.mdpi.com/2218-273X/13/1/28, doi:10.3390/biom13010028.

[221] Saul R. Powell. The Antioxidant Properties of Zinc. *The Journal of Nutrition*, 130(5):1447S–1454S, 2000. URL: https://www.sc

iencedirect.com/science/article/pii/S0022316622141039, doi:https://doi.org/10.1093/jn/130.5.1447S.

[222] Ananda S. Prasad, Bin Bao, Frances W.J. Beck, Omer Kucuk, and Fazlul H. Sarkar. Antioxidant effect of zinc in humans. *Free Radical Biology and Medicine*, 37(8):1182–1190, 2004. URL: https://www.sciencedirect.com/science/article/pii/S0891584904005465, doi:https://doi.org/10.1016/j.freeradbiomed.2004.07.007.

[223] Christopher J. Stadtherr. Nutritional bioavailability – zinc: Revitalize Metabolic Health. Jan 2024. URL: https://revitalizemetabolichealth.com/nutritional-bioavailability-zinc/.

[224] Maria Maares and Hajo Haase. A Guide to Human Zinc Absorption: General Overview and Recent Advances of In Vitro Intestinal Models. *Nutrients*, 2020. URL: https://www.mdpi.com/2072-6643/12/3/762, doi:10.3390/nu12030762.

[225] Kenneth H. Brown, Sara E. Wuehler, and Jan M. Peerson. The Importance of Zinc in Human Nutrition and Estimation of the Global Prevalence of Zinc Deficiency. *Food and Nutrition Bulletin*, 22(2):113–125, 2001. URL: https://doi.org/10.1177/156482 650102200201, arXiv:https://doi.org/10.1177/156482650102200201, doi:10.1177/156482650102200201.

[226] Holly E. Clarke, Neda S. Akhavan, Taylor A. Behl, Michael J. Ormsbee, and Robert C. Hickner. Effect of Creatine Monohydrate Supplementation on Macro- and Microvascular Endothelial Function in Older Adults: A Pilot Study. *Nutrients*, 2025. URL: https://www.mdpi.com/2072-6643/17/1/58, doi:10.3390/nu17010058.

[227] Adrian Aron, Eryn J. Landrum, Adam D. Schneider, Megan Via, Logan Evans, and Eric S. Rawson. Effects of acute creatine supplementation on cardiac and vascular responses in older men; a randomized controlled trial. *Clinical Nutrition ESPEN*, 63:557–563, Oct 2024. doi:10.1016/j.clnesp.2024.07.008.

[228] Annamaria Del Franco, Giuseppe Ambrosio, Laura Baroncelli, Tommaso Pizzorusso, Andrea Barison, Iacopo Olivotto, Fabio A. Recchia, Carlo M. Lombardi, Marco Metra, Yu F. Ferrari Chen, Claudio Passino, Michele Emdin, and Giuseppe Vergaro. Creatine deficiency and heart failure. *Heart Failure Reviews*, 27(5):1605–1616, Sep 2022. URL: https://doi.org/10.1007/s10741-021-10173-y, doi:10.1007/s10741-021-10173-y.

[229] Frank M. Sacks, Laura P. Svetkey, William M. Vollmer, Lawrence J. Appel, George A. Bray, David Harsha, Eva Obarzanek, Paul R. Conlin, Edgar R. Miller, Denise G. Simons-Morton, Njeri Karanja, Pao-Hwa Lin, Mikel Aickin, Marlene M. Most-Windhauser, Thomas J. Moore, Michael A. Proschan, and Jeffrey A. Cutler. Effects on Blood Pressure of Reduced Dietary Sodium and the Dietary Approaches to Stop Hypertension (DASH) Diet. *New England Journal of Medicine*, 344(1):3–10, 2001. URL: https://www.nejm.org/doi/full/10.1056/NEJM200101043440101, arXiv:https://www.nejm.org/doi/pdf/10.1056/NEJM200101043440101, doi:10.1056/NEJM200101043440101.

[230] Allison W. Peng, Lawrence J. Appel, Noel T. Mueller, Olive Tang, Edgar R. Miller III, and Stephen P. Juraschek. Effects of sodium intake on postural lightheadedness: Results from the DASH-sodium trial. *The Journal of Clinical Hypertension*, 21(3):355–362, 2019. URL: https://onlinelibrary.wiley.com/doi/abs/10.1111/jch.13 487, arXiv:https://onlinelibrary.wiley.com/doi/pdf/10.1111/jch.13487, doi:https://doi.org/10.1111/jch.13487.

[231] Paul Belany, Madison L Kackley, Songzhu Zhao, Bjorn Kluwe, Alex Buga, Christopher D Crabtree, Divya Nedungadi, David Kline, Guy Brock, Orlando P Simonetti, Jeff S Volek, and Joshua J Joseph. Effects of Hypocaloric Low-Fat, Ketogenic, and Ketogenic and Ketone Supplement Diets on Aldosterone and Renin. *The Journal of Clinical Endocrinology & Metabolism*,

108(7):1727–1739, 01 2023. URL: https://doi.org/10.1210/
clinem/dgad009, arXiv:https://academic.oup.com/jcem/article-
pdf/108/7/1727/50604599/dgad009.pdf,
doi:10.1210/clinem/dgad009.

[232] Anna Hernández. Adipose tissue: What is it, location, function, and
more. URL: https://www.osmosis.org/answers/adipose-tissue.

[233] David S. Ludwig and Cara B. Ebbeling. The Carbohydrate-Insulin
Model of Obesity: Beyond "Calories In, Calories Out". *JAMA Internal
Medicine*, 178(8):1098–1103, 08 2018. URL: https://doi.org/10.1001/
jamainternmed.2018.2933, doi:10.1001/jamainternmed.2018.2933.

[234] Sebastian D. Parlee, Stephen I. Lentz, Hiroyuki Mori, and Ormond A.
MacDougald. Chapter Six - Quantifying Size and Number of
Adipocytes in Adipose Tissue. In Ormond A. Macdougald, editor,
Methods of Adipose Tissue Biology, Part A, volume 537 of Methods
in Enzymology, pages 93–122. Academic Press, 2014. URL: https://
www.sciencedirect.com/science/article/pii/B9780124116191000069,
doi:https://doi.org/10.1016/B978-0-12-411619-1.00006-9.

[235] M. Lafontan. Adipose tissue and adipocyte dysregulation. *Diabetes
& Metabolism*, 40(1):16–28, 2014. URL: https://www.scienc
edirect.com/science/article/pii/S1262363613001614,
doi:https://doi.org/10.1016/j.diabet.2013.08.002.

[236] Eric S. Freedland. Role of a critical visceral adipose tissue threshold
(cvatt) in metabolic syndrome: implications for controlling dietary
carbohydrates: a review. *Nutrition & Metabolism*, 1(1):12, Nov 2004.
URL: https://doi.org/10.1186/1743-7075-1-12, doi:10.1186/1743-
7075-1-12.

[237] Maggie S. Burhans, Derek K. Hagman, Jessica N. Kuzma,
Kelsey A. Schmidt, and Mario Kratz. *Contribution of Adipose
Tissue Inflammation to the Development of Type 2 Diabetes
Mellitus*, chapter, pages 1–58. John Wiley & Sons, Ltd, 2018. URL:

https://onlinelibrary.wiley.com/doi/abs/10.1002/cphy.c170040, arXiv:https://onlinelibrary.wiley.com/doi/pdf/10.1002/cphy.c170040, doi:https://doi.org/10.1002/cphy.c170040.

[238] Yvonne Döring, Emiel P. C. van der Vorst, and Christian Weber. Targeting immune cell recruitment in atherosclerosis. *Nature Reviews Cardiology*, 21(11):824–840, Nov 2024. URL: https://doi.org/10.103 8/s41569-024-01023-z, doi:10.1038/s41569-024-01023-z.

[239] Merla J. Hubler and Arion J. Kennedy. Role of lipids in the metabolism and activation of immune cells. *The Journal of Nutritional Biochemistry*, 34:1–7, 2016. URL: https://www.scienced irect.com/science/article/pii/S0955286315003368, doi:https://doi.org/10.1016/j.jnutbio.2015.11.002.

[240] Lachlan Mitchell, Stuart B. Murray, Stephen Cobley, Daniel Hackett, Janelle Gifford, Louise Capling, and Helen O'Connor. Muscle dysmorphia symptomatology and associated psychological features in bodybuilders and non-bodybuilder resistance trainers: a systematic review and meta-analysis. *Sports Medicine*, 47(2):233–259, Feb 2017. URL: https://doi.org/10.1007/s40279-016-0564-3, doi:10.1007/s40279-016-0564-3.

[241] M Vecchiato, M Da Col, G Berton, S Palermi, A Aghi, A Ermolao, J Niebauer, J Drezner, and D Neunhaeuserer. Mortality risk in bodybuilding: a call for action to promote safe sport participation. *European Journal of Preventive Cardiology*, 31(Supplement_1):zwae175.277, 06 2024. URL: https://doi.org/10.1093/eurjpc/zwa e175.277, arXiv:https://academic.oup.com/eurjpc/article-pdf/31/Supplement_1/zwae175.277/58221327/zwae175.277.pdf, doi:10.1093/eurjpc/zwae175.277.

[242] Benjamin M. Weisenthal, Christopher A. Beck, Michael D. Maloney, Kenneth E. DeHaven, and Brian D. Giordano. Injury

Rate and Patterns Among CrossFit Athletes. *Orthopaedic Journal of Sports Medicine*, 2(4):2325967114531177, 2014. PMID: 26535325. URL: https://doi.org/10.1177/23259671 1 4 5 3 1 1 77, arXiv:https://doi.org/10.1177/2325967114531177, doi:10.1177/2325967114531177.

[243] Reece Doughty. The danger of high intensity exercise: a case of CrossFit® related rhabdomyolysis. *Proceedings of UCLA Health*, 2017.

[244] Pamodi Kodikara, Rowan Walker, and Scott Wilson. Renal physiology and kidney injury during intense (CrossFit®) exercise. *Internal Medicine Journal*, 53(7):1180–1187, 2023. URL: https://onlinelibrary.wiley.com/doi/abs/10.1111/imj.15667, arXiv:https://onlinelibrary.wiley.com/doi/pdf/10.1111/imj.15667, doi:https://doi.org/10.1111/imj.15667.

[245] Mirwais Mehrab, Robert Kaspar Wagner, Gwendolyn Vuurberg, Vincent Gouttebarge, Robert-Jan de Vos, and Nina Maria Mathijssen. Risk factors for musculoskeletal injury in CrossFit: A systematic review. *International Journal of Sports Medicine*, 44(04):247–257, Sep 2022. doi:10.1055/a-1953-6317.

[246] By Greg Glassman. CrossFit Induced Rhabdo. URL: https://web.arch ive.org/web/20081101095058/http://journal.crossfit.com/2005/10/c rossfit-induced-rhabdo-by-gre.tpl.

[247] Rob Eley. Explainer: What is rhabdomyolysis and what's its connection to CrossFit? Feb 2025. URL: https://theconversation. com/explainer-what-is-rhabdomyolysis-and-whats-its-connection-t o-crossfit-75623.

[248] Toshio Moritani. Neuromuscular adaptations during the acquisition of muscle strength, power and motor tasks. *Journal of Biomechanics*, 26:95–107, 1993. Proceedings of the XIIIth Congress of the International Society of Biomechanics. URL: https://www.scie

ncedirect.com/science/article/pii/002192909390082P,
doi:https://doi.org/10.1016/0021-9290(93)90082-P.

[249] Brett & Kate McKay. Legendary bodybuilder Mike Mentzer's Heavy Duty Method for maximum muscle growth. Mar 2024. URL: https://www.artofmanliness.com/health-fitness/fitness/mike-mentzer-heavy-duty.

[250] Juan Carlos Cassano and Conor Heffernan. Golden paradox. Feb 2025. URL: https://sportrxiv.org/index.php/server/preprint/view/513, doi:10.51224/srxiv.513.

[251] Robert Winker, Alfred Barth, Daniela Bidmon, Ivo Ponocny, Michael Weber, Otmar Mayr, David Robertson, André Diedrich, Richard Maier, Alex Pilger, Paul Haber, and Hugo W. Rüdiger. Endurance Exercise Training in Orthostatic Intolerance. *Hypertension*, 45(3):391–398, 2005. URL: https://www.ahajournals.org/doi/abs/10.1161/01.HYP.0000156540.25707.af, doi:10.1161/01.HYP.0000156540.25707.af.

[252] Darren P. Casey and Emma C. Hart. Cardiovascular function in humans during exercise: role of the muscle pump. *The Journal of Physiology*, 586(21):5045–5046, October 2008. URL: http://dx.doi.org/10.1113/jphysiol.2008.162123, doi:10.1113/jphysiol.2008.162123.

[253] Michelle M. Masterson, Amy L. Morgan, Christine E. Multer, and Daniel Cipriani. The role of lower leg muscle activity in blood pressure maintenance of older adults. *Chapman University Digital Commons*, 2006. URL: https://digitalcommons.chapman.edu/pt_articles/40/.

[254] Johannes J. van Lieshout, Frank Pott, Per Lav Madsen, Jeroen van Goudoever, and Niels H. Secher. Muscle Tensing During Standing . *Stroke*, 32(7):1546–1551, 2001. URL: https://www.ahajournals.org/doi/abs/10.1161/01.STR.32.7.1546,

arXiv:https://www.ahajournals.org/doi/pdf/10.1161/01.STR.32.7.1546, doi:10.1161/01.STR.32.7.1546.

[255] Anthony W. Baross, Jonathan D. Wiles, and Ian L. Swaine. Effects of the Intensity of Leg Isometric Training on the Vasculature of Trained and Untrained Limbs and Resting Blood Pressure in Middle-Aged Men. *International Journal of Vascular Medicine*, 2012(1):964697, 2012. URL: h t t p s : //onlinelibrary.wiley.com/doi/abs/10.1155/2012/964697, arXiv:https://onlinelibrary.wiley.com/doi/pdf/10.1155/2012/964697, doi:https://doi.org/10.1155/2012/964697.

[256] Kyle H. Moore, Hayley A. Murphy, and Eric M. George. The glycocalyx: a central regulator of vascular function. *American Journal of Physiology-Regulatory, Integrative and Comparative Physiology*, 320(4):R508–R518, 2021. PMID: 33501896. URL: h t t p s : / / d o i . o r g / 1 0 . 1 1 5 2 / a j p r e g u . 0 0 3 4 0 . 2 0 20, arXiv:https://doi.org/10.1152/ajpregu.00340.2020, doi:10.1152/ajpregu.00340.2020.

[257] Yu Yao, Aleksandr Rabodzey, and Jr. Dewey, C. Forbes. Glycocalyx modulates the motility and proliferative response of vascular endothelium to fluid shear stress. *American Journal of Physiology-Heart and Circulatory Physiology*, 293(2):H1023–H1030, August 2007. URL: http://dx.doi.org/10.1152/ajpheart.00162.2007, doi:10.1152/ajpheart.00162.2007.

[258] Kyle H. Moore, Hayley A. Murphy, and Eric M. George. The glycocalyx: a central regulator of vascular function. *American Journal of Physiology-Regulatory, Integrative and Comparative Physiology*, 320(4):R508–R518, April 2021. PMID: 33501896. URL: http://dx.doi.org/10.1152/ajpregu.00340.2020, doi:10.1152/ajpregu.00340.2020.

[259] Maria Angela Incalza, Rossella D'Oria, Annalisa Natalicchio, Sebastio Perrini, Luigi Laviola, and Francesco Giorgino. Oxidative

stress and reactive oxygen species in endothelial dysfunction associated with cardiovascular and metabolic diseases. *Vascular Pharmacology*, 100:1–19, January 2018. URL: http://dx.doi.org/1 0.1016/j.vph.2017.05.005, doi:10.1016/j.vph.2017.05.005.

[260] Jing Qu, Yue Cheng, Wenchao Wu, Lixing Yuan, and Xiaojing Liu. Glycocalyx Impairment in Vascular Disease: Focus on Inflammation. *Frontiers in Cell and Developmental Biology*, September 2021. URL: http://dx.doi.org/10.3389/fcell.2021.730621, doi:10.3389/fcell.2021.730621.

[261] Ryo Uchimido, Eric P. Schmidt, and Nathan I. Shapiro. The glycocalyx: a novel diagnostic and therapeutic target in sepsis. *Critical Care*, January 2019. URL: http://dx.doi.org/10.1186/s13 054-018-2292-6, doi:10.1186/s13054-018-2292-6.

[262] Daniel Chappell and Matthias Jacob. Role of the glycocalyx in fluid management: Small things matter. *Best Practice & Research Clinical Anaesthesiology*, 28(3):227–234, September 2014. URL: http://dx.doi.org/10.1016/j.bpa.2014.06.003, doi:10.1016/j.bpa.2014.06.003.

[263] Alexandra Puchwein-Schwepcke, Orsolya Genzel-Boroviczény, and Claudia Nussbaum. The Endothelial Glycocalyx: Physiology and Pathology in Neonates, Infants and Children. *Frontiers in Cell and Developmental Biology*, September 2021. URL: http://dx.doi.org/10. 3389/fcell.2021.733557, doi:10.3389/fcell.2021.733557.

[264] Zhengping Hu, Issahy Cano, and Patricia A. D'Amore. Update on the Role of the Endothelial Glycocalyx in Angiogenesis and Vascular Inflammation. *Frontiers in Cell and Developmental Biology*, August 2021. URL: http://dx.doi.org/10.3389/fcell.2021.734276, doi:10.3389/fcell.2021.734276.

[265] Nur Arfian, Wiwit Ananda Wahyu Setyaningsih, Muhammad Mansyur Romi, and Dwi Cahyani Ratna Sari. Heparanase

upregulation from adipocyte associates with inflammation and endothelial injury in diabetic condition. *BMC Proceedings*, December 2019. URL: http://dx.doi.org/10.1186/s12919-019-0181-x, doi:10.1186/s12919-019-0181-x.

[266] Bogna Gryszczyńska, Magdalena Budzyń, Beata Begier-Krasińska, Angelika Osińska, Maciej Boruczkowski, Mariusz Kaczmarek, Alicja Bukowska, Maria Iskra, and Magdalena Paulina Kasprzak. Association between Advanced Glycation End Products, Soluble RAGE Receptor, and Endothelium Dysfunction, Evaluated by Circulating Endothelial Cells and Endothelial Progenitor Cells in Patients with Mild and Resistant Hypertension. *International Journal of Molecular Sciences*, 20(16):3942, August 2019. URL: http://dx.doi .org/10.3390/ijms20163942, doi:10.3390/ijms20163942.

[267] Jing Liu, Shuo Pan, Xiqiang Wang, Zhongwei Liu, and Yong Zhang. Role of advanced glycation end products in diabetic vascular injury: molecular mechanisms and therapeutic perspectives. *European Journal of Medical Research*, December 2023. URL: http: //dx.doi.org/10.1186/s40001-023-01431-w, doi:10.1186/s40001-023-01431-w.

[268] Slava Rom, Nathan A. Heldt, Sachin Gajghate, Alecia Seliga, Nancy L. Reichenbach, and Yuri Persidsky. Hyperglycemia and advanced glycation end products disrupt BBB and promote occludin and claudin-5 protein secretion on extracellular microvesicles. *Scientific Reports*, April 2020. URL: http://dx.doi.org/10.1038/s4159 8-020-64349-x, doi:10.1038/s41598-020-64349-x.

[269] Daniel R. Potter, John Jiang, and Edward R. Damiano. The Recovery Time Course of the Endothelial Cell Glycocalyx In Vivo and Its Implications In Vitro. *Circulation Research*, 104(11):1318–1325, June 2009. URL: http://dx.doi.org/10.1161/CIRCRESAHA.108. 191585, doi:10.1161/circresaha.108.191585.

[270] Paula Franceković and Lasse Gliemann. Endothelial Glycocalyx Preservation—Impact of Nutrition and Lifestyle. *Nutrients*, 15(11):2573, May 2023. URL: http://dx.doi.org/10.3390/nu15112573, doi:10.3390/nu15112573.

[271] Mayo Clinic. Propafenone (Oral Route) - Description and Side Effects. Accessed: 2025-05-18. URL: https://www.mayoclinic.org/drugs-sup plements/propafenone-oral-route/description/drg-20065687#drug-s ide-effects.

[272] MedlinePlus. Propafenone: Side Effects. Accessed: 2025-05-18. URL: https://medlineplus.gov/druginfo/meds/a698002.html#sid e-effects.

[273] WebMD. Propafenone (Rythmol) - Uses, Side Effects, and MorePropafenone (Rythmol) - Uses, Side Effects, and More. Accessed: 2025-05-18. URL: https://www.webmd.com/drugs/2/drug -8838-4070/propafenone-oral/propafenone-oral/details.

[274] Mayo Clinic. Aspirin (oral route). Accessed: 2025-05-18. URL: https: //www.mayoclinic.org/drugs-supplements/aspirin-oral-route/descrip tion/drg-20152665.

[275] Drugs.com. Aspirin (oral route). Accessed: 2025-05-18. URL: https: //www.mayoclinic.org/drugs-supplements/aspirin-oral-route/descrip tion/drg-20152665.

[276] WebMD. Aspirin (Bayer, Vazalore, and others) - Uses, Side Effects, and More. Accessed: 2025-05-18. URL: https://www.webmd.com/dr ugs/2/drug-21688/baby-aspirin-oral/details.

[277] Peiqiu Zheng, Xing Wang, Tao Guo, Wei Gao, Qiang Huang, Jie Yang, Hui Gao, and Qian Liu. Cardiac troponin as a prognosticator of mortality in patients with sepsis: A systematic review and meta-analysis. *Immunity, Inflammation and Disease*, September 2023. URL: http://dx.doi.org/10.1002/iid3.1014, doi:10.1002/iid3.1014.

[278] Franklin Dexter, Alex Macario, Rodney D. Traub, Margaret Hopwood, and David A. Lubarsky. An Operating Room Scheduling Strategy to Maximize the Use of Operating Room Block Time. *Anesthesia & Analgesia*, 89(1):7–20, July 1999. URL: http://dx.doi.org/10.1213 /00000539-199907000-00003, doi:10.1213/00000539-199907000-00003.

[279] Ileo-Caecal Resection.

[280] Cleveland Clinic medical professional. Anastomosis: Definition, types & procedure. Mar 2025. URL: https://my.clevelandclinic.o rg/health/treatments/24035-anastomosis.

[281] Claire Pilet, Florentine Tandzi-Tonleu, Emmanuel Lagarde, Cédric Gil-Jardiné, Michel Galinski, and Sylviane Lafont. Feelings of Patients Admitted to the Emergency Department. *Healthcare*, 2025. URL: https://www.mdpi.com/2227-9032/13/5/500, doi:10.3390/healthcare13050500.

[282] Madhukar Jaygopal, Sandeep Jain, Sameer Malhotra, Anoop Purkayastha, and Shreya Singhal. Factors affecting stress levels in attendants accompanying patients to emergency department. *Journal of Emergencies, Trauma, and Shock*, 15(3):116–123, Jul 2022. doi:10.4103/jets.jets_156_21.

[283] Laszlo Irsay, Viorela Mihaela Ciortea, Theodor Popa, Madalina Gabriela Iliescu, and Alina Deniza Ciubean. Exploring the Connections between Medical Rehabilitation, Faith and Spirituality. *Healthcare*, 2024. URL: https://www.mdpi.com/2227-9032/12/12/12 02, doi:10.3390/healthcare12121202.

[284] The influence of Faith on Trauma Recovery.

[285] Nahathai Wongpakaran, Sirilux Klaychaiya, Chompimaksorn Panuspanudechdamrong, Natapoom Techasomboon, Pookit Chaipinchana, Justin DeMaranville, Zsuzsanna Kövi, and Tinakon

Wongpakaran. A comparative study of the impact of meditation and buddhist five precepts on stress and depression between older adults and younger adults. *Scientific Reports*, 15(1):15739, May 2025. URL: https://doi.org/10.1038/s41598-025-99430-w, doi:10.1038/s41598-025-99430-w.

[286] Megan E. L. Brown, Alexander MacLellan, William Laughey, Usmaan Omer, Ghita Himmi, Tim LeBon, and Gabrielle M. Finn. Can stoic training develop medical student empathy and resilience? a mixed-methods study. *BMC Medical Education*, 22(1):340, May 2022. URL: https://doi.org/10.1186/s12909-022-03391-x, doi:10.1186/s12909-022-03391-x.

[287] Timothy R. Matsuura, Patrycja Puchalska, Peter A. Crawford, and Daniel P. Kelly. Ketones and the Heart: Metabolic Principles and Therapeutic Implications. *Circulation Research*, 132(7):882–898, 2023. URL: https://www.ahajournals.org/doi/abs/10.1161/CIRCRESAHA.123.321872, doi:10.1161/CIRCRESAHA.123.321872.

[288] Inna Sokolova. Mitochondrial Adaptations to Variable Environments and Their Role in Animals' Stress Tolerance. *Integrative and Comparative Biology*, 58(3):519–531, April 2018. URL: http://dx.doi.org/10.1093/icb/icy017, doi:10.1093/icb/icy017.

[289] Christopher F. Bennett, Pedro Latorre-Muro, and Pere Puigserver. Mechanisms of mitochondrial respiratory adaptation. *Nature Reviews Molecular Cell Biology*, 23(12):817–835, July 2022. URL: http://dx.doi.org/10.1038/s41580-022-00506-6, doi:10.1038/s41580-022-00506-6.

[290] Lucia-Doina Popov. Mitochondrial biogenesis: An update. *Journal of Cellular and Molecular Medicine*, 24(9):4892–4899, April 2020. URL: http://dx.doi.org/10.1111/jcmm.15194, doi:10.1111/jcmm.15194.

[291] Stephane Arques and Pierre Ambrosi. Human Serum Albumin in the Clinical Syndrome of Heart Failure. *Journal of Cardiac Failure*, 17(6):451–458, June 2011. URL: http://dx.doi.org/10.1016/j.cardfail.2011.02.010, doi:10.1016/j.cardfail.2011.02.010.

[292] Lawrence Baudendistel, Thomas E. Dahms, and Donald L. Kaminski. The effect of albumin on extravascular lung water in animals and patients with low-pressure pulmonary edema. *Journal of Surgical Research*, 33(4):285–293, October 1982. URL: http://dx.doi.org/1 0.1016/0022-4804(82)90041-5, doi:10.1016/0022-4804(82)90041-5.

[293] Hesham R. Omar, Mehdi Mirsaeidi, Rania Rashad, Hatem Hassaballa, Garett Enten, Engy Helal, Devanand Mangar, and Enrico M. Camporesi. Association of Serum Albumin and Severity of Pulmonary Embolism. *Medicina*, 56(1):26, January 2020. URL: http://dx.doi.org /10.3390/medicina56010026, doi:10.3390/medicina56010026.

[294] Rajat N Moman, Nishant Gupta, and Matthew Varacallo. Physiology, albumin. *StatPearls [Internet].*, 2017. URL: https://www.ncbi.nlm.n ih.gov/books/NBK459198/.

[295] Christian Ephata Issangya, David Msuya, Kondo Chilonga, Ayesiga Herman, Elichilia Shao, Febronia Shirima, Elifaraja Naman, Henry Mkumbi, Jeremia Pyuza, Emmanuel Mtui, Leah Anku Sanga, Seif Abdul, Beatrice John Leyaro, and Samuel Chugulu. Perioperative serum albumin as a predictor of adverse outcomes in abdominal surgery: prospective cohort hospital based study in northern tanzania. *BMC Surgery*, 20(1):155, Jul 2020. URL: https://doi.org/10.1186/s1 2893-020-00820-w, doi:10.1186/s12893-020-00820-w.

[296] Catharina Müller, Anton Stift, Stanislaus Argeny, Michael Bergmann, Michael Gnant, Sebastian Marolt, Lukas Unger, and Stefan Riss. Delta albumin is a better prognostic marker for complications following laparoscopic intestinal resection for crohn's disease than

albumin alone - A retrospective cohort study. *PLOS ONE*, Nov 2018. doi:10.1371/journal.pone.0206911.

[297] Kang Hu, Ke Tan, Quanzhen Shang, Chao Li, Zhe Zhang, Bin Huang, Song Zhao, Fan Li, Anping Zhang, Chunxue Li, Baohua Liu, and Weidong Tong. Relative decline in serum albumin help to predict anastomotic leakage for female patients following sphincter-preserving rectal surgery. *BMC Surgery*, 23(1):38, Feb 2023. URL: https://doi.org/10.1186/s12893-023-01923-w, doi:10.1186/s12893-023-01923-w.

[298] Cole A. Nipper, Kelvin Lim, Carlos Riveros, Enshuo Hsu, Sanjana Ranganathan, Jiaqiong Xu, Michael Brooks, Nestor Esnaola, Zachary Klaassen, Angela Jerath, Amanda Arrington, Christopher J. D. Wallis, and Raj Satkunasivam. The Association between Serum Albumin and Post-Operative Outcomes among Patients Undergoing Common Surgical Procedures: An Analysis of a Multi-Specialty Surgical Cohort from the National Surgical Quality Improvement Program (NSQIP). *Journal of Clinical Medicine*, 2022. URL: https://www.mdpi.com/2077-0383/11/21/6543, doi:10.3390/jcm11216543.

[299] Hong Xu, Li Liu, Jinwei Xie, Duan Wang, Zeyu Huang, and Zongke Zhou. A pre-operative high-protein diet can improve the serum albumin levels of patients undergoing total knee arthroplasty. *Chinese Medical Journal*, 136(4):491–493, Feb 2023. doi:10.1097/cm9.0000000000002209.

[300] Daniel R Moore, Meghann J Robinson, Jessica L Fry, Jason E Tang, Elisa I Glover, Sarah B Wilkinson, Todd Prior, Mark A Tarnopolsky, and Stuart M Phillips. Ingested protein dose response of muscle and albumin protein synthesis after resistance exercise in young men. *The American Journal of Clinical Nutrition*, 89(1):161–168, 2009. URL: https://www.sciencedirect.com/science/article/pii/S0002916523239209, doi:https://doi.org/10.3945/ajcn.2008.26401.

[301] Arik Sheinenzon, Mona Shehadeh, Regina Michelis, Ety Shaoul, and Ohad Ronen. Serum albumin levels and inflammation. *International Journal of Biological Macromolecules*, 184:857–862, 2021. URL: ht tps://www.sciencedirect.com/science/article/pii/S014181302101369 6, doi:https://doi.org/10.1016/j.ijbiomac.2021.06.140.

[302] Laetitia Dou and Noémie Jourde-Chiche. Endothelial Toxicity of High Glucose and its by-Products in Diabetic Kidney Disease. *Toxins*, 11(10):578, October 2019. URL: http://dx.doi.org/10.3390/toxins111 00578, doi:10.3390/toxins11100578.

[303] Takashi Himoto and Tsutomu Masaki. Associations between Zinc Deficiency and Metabolic Abnormalities in Patients with Chronic Liver Disease. *Nutrients*, 10(1):88, January 2018. URL: http://dx.d oi.org/10.3390/nu10010088, doi:10.3390/nu10010088.

[304] Panu K. Luukkonen, Sylvie Dufour, Kun Lyu, Xian-Man Zhang, Antti Hakkarainen, Tiina E. Lehtimäki, Gary W. Cline, Kitt Falk Petersen, Gerald I. Shulman, and Hannele Yki-Järvinen. Effect of a ketogenic diet on hepatic steatosis and hepatic mitochondrial metabolism in nonalcoholic fatty liver disease. *Proceedings of the National Academy of Sciences*, 117(13):7347–7354, March 2020. URL: http://dx.doi.org /10.1073/pnas.1922344117, doi:10.1073/pnas.1922344117.

[305] Celeste C. Finnerty, Nigel Tapiwa Mabvuure, Arham Ali, Rosemary A. Kozar, and David N. Herndon. The Surgically Induced Stress Response. *Journal of Parenteral and Enteral Nutrition*, September 2013. URL: http://dx.doi.org/10.1177/014860711349611 7, doi:10.1177/0148607113496117.

[306] Moto Kashiwabara, Masao Miyashita, Tsutomu Nomura, Hiroshi Makino, Takeshi Matsutani, Chol Kim, Shinhiro Takeda, Kiyohiko Yamashita, Irshad H. Chaudry, and Takashi Tajiri. Surgical Trauma-Induced Adrenal Insufficiency is Associated with Postoperative Inflammatory Responses. *Journal of Nippon Medical School*,

74(4):274–283, 2007. URL: http://dx.doi.org/10.1272/jnms.74.274, doi:10.1272/jnms.74.274.

[307] Jun Tian and Yan Li. Comparative effects of vitamin C on the effects of local anesthetics ropivacaine, bupivacaine, and lidocaine on human chondrocytes. *Brazilian Journal of Anesthesiology (English Edition)*, 66(1):29–36, January 2016. URL: http://dx.doi.org/10.1016/j.bjane.2 015.01.006, doi:10.1016/j.bjane.2015.01.006.

[308] Yiying Zhang, Chuxiong Pan, Xu Wu, Yuanlin Dong, Deborah J. Culley, Gregory Crosby, Tianzuo Li, and Zhongcong Xie. Different effects of anesthetic isoflurane on caspase-3 activation and cytosol cytochrome c levels between mice neural progenitor cells and neurons. *Frontiers in Cellular Neuroscience*, 2014. URL: http://dx.doi.org/10. 3389/fncel.2014.00014, doi:10.3389/fncel.2014.00014.

[309] Ying Cheng, Linda He, Vidhya Prasad, Shuang Wang, and Richard J. Levy. Anesthesia-Induced Neuronal Apoptosis in the Developing Retina. *Anesthesia & Analgesia*, 121(5):1325–1335, November 2015. URL: http://dx.doi.org/10.1213/ANE.0000000000000714, doi:10.1213/ane.0000000000000714.

[310] Allison J. Rao, Tyler R. Johnston, Alex H.S. Harris, R. Lane Smith, and John G. Costouros. Inhibition of Chondrocyte and Synovial Cell Death After Exposure to Commonly Used Anesthetics. *The American Journal of Sports Medicine*, 42(1):50–58, October 2013. URL: http://dx.doi.org/10.1177/0363546513507426, doi:10.1177/0363546513507426.

[311] Nicholas N. DePhillipo, Zachary S. Aman, Mitchell I. Kennedy, J.P. Begley, Gilbert Moatshe, and Robert F. LaPrade. Efficacy of Vitamin C Supplementation on Collagen Synthesis and Oxidative Stress After Musculoskeletal Injuries: A Systematic Review. *Orthopaedic Journal of Sports Medicine*, October 2018. URL: http://dx.doi.org/10.1177/2 325967118804544, doi:10.1177/2325967118804544.

[312] Luana Dias Campos, Valfredo de Almeida Santos Junior, Júlia Demuner Pimentel, Gabriel Lusi Fernandes Carregã, and Cinthia Baú Betim Cazarin. Collagen supplementation in skin and orthopedic diseases: A review of the literature. *Heliyon*, 9(4):e14961, April 2023. URL: http://dx.doi.org/10.1016/j.heliyon.2023.e14961, doi:10.1016/j.heliyon.2023.e14961.

[313] H.J.M. de Kok. Is there an overlap between irritable bowel syndrome and appendicopathy syndrome? A new theory. *Medical Hypotheses*, 75(6):501–504, December 2010. URL: http://dx.doi.org/10.1016/j.m ehy.2010.07.005, doi:10.1016/j.mehy.2010.07.005.

[314] Lars Ivo Partecke, Andrea Thiele, Franziska Schmidt-Wankel, Wolfram Kessler, Michael Wodny, Frank Dombrowski, Claus-Dieter Heidecke, and Wolfram von Bernstorff. Appendicopathy—a clinical and diagnostic dilemma. *International Journal of Colorectal Disease*, 28(8):1081–1089, March 2013. URL: http://dx.doi.org/10.1007/s00 384-013-1677-x, doi:10.1007/s00384-013-1677-x.

[315] Charles C. van Rossem, Kaij Treskes, David L. Loeza, and Anna A. W. van Geloven. Laparoscopic appendectomy for chronic right lower quadrant abdominal pain. *International Journal of Colorectal Disease*, 29(10):1199–1202, July 2014. URL: http://dx.doi.org/10.10 07/s00384-014-1978-8, doi:10.1007/s00384-014-1978-8.

[316] Bartosz Bogielski, Katarzyna Michalczyk, Piotr Głodek, Bartosz Tempka, Wojciech Gębski, and Dominika Stygar. Association between small intestine bacterial overgrowth and psychiatric disorders. *Frontiers in Endocrinology*, October 2024. URL: http://dx.doi.org/10. 3389/fendo.2024.1438066, doi:10.3389/fendo.2024.1438066.

[317] Kuo-Chuan Hung, Yao-Tsung Lin, Kee-Hsin Chen, Li-Kai Wang, Jen-Yin Chen, Ying-Jen Chang, Shao-Chun Wu, Min-Hsien Chiang, and Cheuk-Kwan Sun. The Effect of Perioperative Vitamin C on Postoperative Analgesic Consumption: A Meta-Analysis of

Randomized Controlled Trials. *Nutrients*, 12(10):3109, October 2020. URL: h t tp : / / d x . d o i . o r g / 1 0 . 3 3 9 0 / n u 1 2 1 0 3 1 0 9, doi:10.3390/nu12103109.

[318] Norman Cousins. *Anatomy of an illness as perceived by the patient.* W.W. Norton, 2005.

[319] Kheira Lakhdari. *Conception et Développement d'un Assistant Mobile Intelligent pour le Suivi des Maladies Chroniques.* Thèse de Doctorat en Télécommunication, Université Abou Bekr Belkaid Tlemcen, 2024. Accessed via the Wayback Machine. URL: https://web.archive.org/web/20240911062311/http://dspace.univ-tlemcen.dz/bitstream/112/16100/1/Doc.Tel.Lakhdari.pdf.

INDEX

www.ingramcontent.com/pod-product-compliance
Lightning Source LLC
Chambersburg PA
CBHW060316050426
42449CB00011B/2508